Cynical Acumen

The anarchic guide to clinical medicine

John Larkin

Radcliffe Publishing

Oxford • Seattle

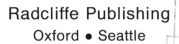

Radcliffe Publishing Ltd
18 Marcham Road
Abingdon
Oxon OX14 1AA
United Kingdom

www.radcliffe-oxford.com
Electronic catalogue and worldwide online ordering facility.

Reprinted 2006

British Library Cataloguing in Publication Data

A catalogue record for this book is available from the British Library.

ISBN 978 1 85775 787 3

Typeset by Aarontype Ltd, Easton, Bristol
Printed and bound by TJ International Ltd, Padstow, Cornwall

Contents

Preface

The plan is for this book to be banned.

In a marketplace stuffed to the gunnels with medical textbooks, surgical textbooks, clinical textbooks ... something is required to set a new volume apart from the others. Something has to catch the eye of the potential reader. In the absence of any superior qualifications, testimonials or indeed literary merit, I have decided that being banned is clearly the best bet. It worked for Jane Birkin (*Je t'aime moi non plus*[1]), for *Frankie Goes to Hollywood* and – of course, most appropriately – for DH Lawrence and Nabokov. *Lady Chatterley's Lover* would have sold no copies at all if it were not for its unavailability, while *Lolita* famously struggled for wider recognition until it was banned by the Paris Police.

It is perhaps unfortunate that the above examples may suggest that this book transcends the accepted boundaries of unbridled sexuality and eroticism for a medical textbook. My apologies for any disappointment. Would that this were the case.[2] While the very use of the word 'eroticism' might indeed be enough to outrage the medical establishment's standards of decency, the target is more one of offending that same establishment with an unacceptable measure of cynicism.

It must be said that the aim is not to cause upset deliberately, but merely finding to my surprise that a candid account of a practical approach to patients and their problems – as well as other practitioners and the problems that *they* cause – is not in keeping with what one would call 'good medical practice'. My hopes in this regard are given a boost by the response to an earlier piece on 'Cynical Acumen' in *Hospital Doctor*. Two weeks after its publication there appeared not a letter but an entire article lambasting my opinions and professing a hope beyond hope that I would never in the future be allowed anywhere near our beloved impressionable student population.

It will be nice to reach a wider audience.

John Larkin
October 2005

---

[1] The added appeal of this surprise 1969 hit record was that no one quite understood what the title was supposed to mean.

[2] An interesting sentence construction which confounds many (*moi non plus*), but which I have always wanted to try out.

About the author

John Larkin is a consultant rheumatologist/physician at the Victoria Infirmary in Glasgow, his arguably irrelevant MD in the clinical pharmacology of epilepsy betraying an eclectic approach to both education and life. An Honorary Senior Clinical Lectureship at Glasgow University and a position as Examiner for the Glasgow College of Physicians and Surgeons lend bogus gravitas to a passionate interest in the practicalities of teaching. His outside interests are legion, but he never allows his work as a practising clinician to interfere with them. He has one wife, three grown-up children and a large number of unpublished stories and scripts.

Acknowledgements

My thanks to Howard McAlpine, Tom Pullar, Fiona McGarry, David Vernon, John-Paul Leach and Helen Dallal for reviewing chapters in their respective specialties. Further thanks to Anna Larkin for help with the illustrations. Also thanks to countless colleagues who have had to tolerate many of the enclosed ramblings over coffee over the years, and to the patients and students who have inspired those ramblings. Further thanks to everyone at Radcliffe Publishing, who took irreverence in their stride, and who all seem very nice, so far.

To
Louie
... and Damian, Des and David ...
... and for Stefan, who thought the Endocrine chapter 'could be longer'.

Introduction

> The purpose of a doctor is to entertain the patient while the disease takes its course ...

The above quote from Voltaire (never considered a great fan of doctors) is often viewed as one of literature's greatest insults to the medical profession (the other being Arthur Conan Doyle). I don't think it is an insult at all. One might suggest a direct comparison with that other famous dictum of a doctor's lot: '... to cure rarely, to relieve often, but to console always ...'[1] What is 'entertainment' if not consoling the patient? I view it as one of my duties to at least try to let the patient enjoy their visit. I admit this is not universally appreciated. Some patients view any attempts at humour as a major insult — a sure giveaway that one is not taking their disease as seriously as one ought to. This observation seems a good time to introduce one of the features of this book, namely:

Cynical Tip No. 1   If a newly referred patient takes offence at a lightly humoured approach to the consultation, they are less likely to have anything wrong with them.[2]

'Cynical Tips' will appear throughout this book. They are highly opinionated, of doubtful authenticity and in no way recommended for impressionable persons about to embark (or recently embarked) upon a career in medicine. They will therefore be clearly flagged by bold print so that they may be avoided with relative ease.

In their defence, I must say that their function includes some effort to deal with the-diagnosis-that-dare-not-speak-its-name. NWWT. It is politically incorrect to suggest that some patients have nothing wrong with them. Once analysed, we can see that in this instance the politically correct are (it pains me to admit) correct. We all have something wrong with us. Many, however, have nothing wrong with them in the area in which they would like us to say they have something wrong. The reasons why they would wish us to make a particular diagnosis may not be obvious, but a number of possibilities might be postulated.

---

[1] Occasionally attributed to Hippocrates, no one seems entirely sure where this comes from. Hence it is never quoted in the same form twice.
[2] It is an entirely different form of cynicism which might make the reader suggest an alternative explanation.

It could be simply financial. Attendance allowances, sick-time off work and retirement on medical grounds might all depend on their having a clear-cut illness that the authorities will recognise. More subtly, the patient's role in their family or personal society may depend on their having some disability/illness which merits physical or emotional help and support. The parent who develops needs as the last chicken threatens to fly the coop is an acknowledged concept in all levels of literature (from *Sons and Lovers* to *Steptoe and Son*), but more subtle examples of role-defining or emotional gain are less well recognised.

Patients may also want a particular diagnosis for psychological reasons; perhaps to avoid the stigma (or self-awareness) of a less welcome one. Fibromyalgia might thus be a more acceptable label than depression. Alternatively, they may simply seek reassurance, exaggerating their symptoms to make sure you take things seriously enough to 'do all the tests' and ensure nothing's missed.

With all these possibilities (and not the slightest mention of 'malingering'), the wonder is that some PC-johnnies will still insist that 'no one would ever make up symptoms'.

The idea of the Cynical Tips is to help identify the times when things may not be all that they seem. They are not ways of 'catching out' the patient so that you can wave your smartness triumphantly under their nose. They are there to help you make the correct diagnosis. Even if we admit that nothing-wrong-with-you[3] does exist, there remains the question of whether it is appropriate to try to spot it. The PC brigade seems to forget that by failing to acknowledge the NWWY scenario, they are obliged to come up with a diagnosis, which will perforce be a *wrong* diagnosis. It doesn't stop there. In order to avoid accusations of inactivity, this leads to wrong treatments (or, at least, unnecessary investigations). Countless patients get recurrent courses of steroids for non-existent asthma. I've seen a man pushed towards renal failure by escalating doses of furosemide, the culprit being an institutional refusal to acknowledge that his worsening dyspnoea might be psychogenic.

As well as avoiding potential toxicity from unnecessary treatments, a willing-ness to assess the veracity of a patient's troubles makes it more likely that you will spot any underlying problem. They may prefer the diagnosis of arthritis to depression,[4] but if the depression is treatable, in the end you may be thanked for 'getting it right'.

A third reason. At some time in the future you may be writing medical reports, appearing in court, perhaps saying this man's back is in perpetual agony, that he can't lift a leg off the bed, that even passive flexion of $10°$ causes excruciating pain. If your 'opposite number' for the defence asks 'so why is it he can sit bolt upright with his legs straight in front of him?', you'll wish you had been aware of this manoeuvre rather than looking a right Charlie. It's all very well being PC, but in court the rule is you tell the whole truth.

The cynical approach doesn't change the default position – that the patient is unwell and what he or she says, goes. It just means that sometimes you may have

---

[3] A more confrontational version of NWWT.

[4] I've never quite understood the stigma associated with depression, perhaps because I believe no intelligent person could ever avoid it (did I write that out loud?). With patients I compare it to diabetes, only in depression you're a bit short of neurotransmitters instead of insulin, '... so if we have to give you some glutamic acid substitute instead of insulin, how is that your fault?'

to look further to find what is actually wrong, so that you can address that. You could say that *cynical acumen* means not making the first diagnosis that comes to mind, but the right one. Then you can try to make it better – because that is, after all, the plan. A cynic isn't someone who 'knows the price of everything and the value of nothing'. He knows fine well the value of everything, but isn't always willing to pay the price.

The cynical approach to doctors and the world of medicine is another thing altogether, but we'll get there ...

Where were we? Oh yeah, Cynical Tips. None of the above justifies actually reading them.

Cynical Tip No. 2 Real examination of a patient is different from examination in an examination.

Attempts will be made to differentiate between what really helps clinically and what you will be required to do so that you pass exams and get a chance to help clinically.[5]

Another feature you will have noticed is a tendency towards the use of footnotes. This is not exclusively designed to irritate the publisher (a happy bonus), but to give the book a more personal feel ... like a bedside teaching session where the tutor goes off at tangents to make unconnected observations about the ways of the world, literature, football or Thai cuisine in the middle of an exposition of the examination of the cranial nerves (lemon grass is *the* thing for testing olfactory function).[6]

This book, you see, is not trying to teach you everything. Indeed, it's not really trying to teach you anything. It won't have huge lists of causes, or effects, or every single manoeuvre you should carry out when examining a particular toe.[7] Instead, it attempts to document what one person gets to know over time, a distillation of all the little observations, tips, personal insights and flashes of genius that I've come up with in 25 years – then padded out so that it fills more than a page. It's not written with a mound of specialist textbooks sitting on the desk. It's not even written at a desk, but in a quiet living-room with Elgar in the background.[8] Occasionally a colleague may be asked for some relaxed confirmation, but only four things in the book have actually been 'looked up' to confirm their correctness.[9] This leads, I believe, to a more flowing (in a jaggy, footnoted sort of way) style to the book. It also no doubt leads to a staggering number of exclusions, doubtful interpretations, and – let's face it – total inaccuracies.

---

[5] Just occasionally they do overlap.

[6] A specific resemblance to bedside teaching – of which I am particularly proud – is the tendency for sections to spend too long giving excessive detail at the beginning, then running out of steam towards the end, as 'coffee' approaches. Again using cranial nerves to illustrate this, you will find the first few invoke pernickety details of their individual assessment, while the lower nerves are lumped together in a morass of fatigue and ennui.

[7] It was brought home to me many years ago that any book purporting to do so required to severely limit its scope ... in my chemistry days at Uni ... finding in the library an 1100-page volume entitled *Formaldehyde*.

[8] The *Jacqueline du Pré*, of course. The *nonpareille* until Radiohead get round to doing a cover.

[9] We may run a competition for readers who are willing to guess which.

Clinical medicine is not a science, but an art. Teaching medicine, in my opinion, is even more so. About a year ago, as my bedside-teaching group filed out murmuring their thanks, the last one added '... thank you ... most entertaining'. It was then that I decided to write this book. As Monsieur Voltaire would say:

> ... the purpose of the medical teacher is to entertain the students while they take their course ...

1

General history and examination

History

'Let the patient tell his story' is the traditional advice – with much to commend it – but also carrying all the trite hallmarks of advice from someone who doesn't actually have to do the biz. Paternalism and political correctness rolled into one. And overstated. You obviously have to give the patient a chance to tell his own story (otherwise there'd be no prospect of later having fun picking holes in it), but he doesn't know what it is you want to know, so it won't always work out.

'So what were you feeling wrong that you came into hospital?'[1]

'Well, my daughter panicked, and she phoned the doctor – but Doctor Brown wasn't in because he's away on holiday, so she spoke to Doctor ... oh ... what's her name? ... she came two years ago ... used to be in that practice in the West End ... what is her name? ... [*I'm sorry, but eventually you just have to say it doesn't matter*] ... and she said we should call an ambulance ...'

'But what were you actually feeling wrong?'

'Well, Doctor ... what *is* her name again? ... [*'yes????'*] thought it might be the same thing as last time ...'

'But what did you actually feel? ...' etc.

Patients do need some nudging, coercing, (teasing?) and direct questions to give you a chance to do your job – which does after all include working out what's wrong with them and trying to make it better. It's an interesting modernism. We would never suggest that a car mechanic/plumber should base his assessment entirely on what you think is important to tell him about your car/central heating (or indeed, if you are a cardiologist, your car central heating) rather than on answers to the questions that *he* wants to ask. Yet the world seems to believe that doctors should conform to this system. It's easy to say that a 'good' doctor should 'let the patient tell their story', but it's also what a lazy doctor will do. Let the patient tell things their way – which will include their relatives', friends' and GP's diagnoses – and just go along with it. Pick a predetermined diagnosis – and stick to it. Saves all that nasty thinking and stuff.

I mentioned relatives and friends.

Time was when a patient would turn up to see their doctor and the two of them would sit down together. A quiet confidential moment, almost intimate, when the patient tells the doctor their most secret problems and he tries his best to solve them. Then somebody realised, quite correctly, that there are times when it would

---

[1] Studiously avoiding the '*Q: What brought you into hospital? A: An ambulance*' routine.

be nice, or helpful, for the patient to have someone 'close to them' as a companion. All very reasonable.

How did it become the norm?

It was always sensible that a young teenage girl – or boy – would be accompanied by their parents. Then older teenagers needed support, and suddenly adult 21-year-old women would turn up with their mummy and daddy to discuss the vagaries of their menstrual cycle. As patients go through their twenties, the father usually drops away (for one reason or another), but mum still turns up, making sure that her baby is well looked after. Then there appears a 'window of competence' around the time of the patient being a young parent, when she is considered able to look after herself,[2] but this is quickly supplanted by her own children reaching pugnacious maturity and turning up[3] to make sure that their mother doesn't get mucked about by those pesky doctors.[4]

But we don't take this lying down. The clinic nurse – no longer required as the patient's representative, confidante and general emotional dogsbody – now becomes the doctor's back-up. A chaperone for his benefit rather than the patient's, not just for the examination but as a witness to any tricky conversations where he may need some third party's sworn statement on whether he was rude, opinionated, uninterested, arrogant (the worst) or just plain untidy in his appearance.[5]

Escalation is the name of the game as the patient's relatives are obliged to reply in kind (two daughters are particularly tricky, especially if one is from Canada). Add in the occasional medical or nursing student and our confidential little consulting room is fit to burst with seething humanity, generating an atmosphere not entirely conducive to good medicine even before somebody sends out for pizza.

And that's just relatives. Friends are a whole new ball game ...

It's not right.

But it's emblazoned on tablets of plastic in 'the Patient's Charter',[6] so you're gonna hafta live with it.

Examination

This will be dealt with in the individual chapters.

Just remember one thing.

Whether the patient is a patient in real life, or a patient in an exam, they are a human being. A person.

At some point, they'll be you.

---

[2] Though not the four-year-old who runs about the consulting-room juggling syringes and needles.

[3] '... and isn't that where you used to keep the syringes? ...'

[4] 'You must remember, doctor ... this is my *mother* we're talking about. She may be just a patient to you but just remember, she is *my mother*.' Yes. But perhaps ... just perhaps you could remember that she's **not mine**. Yes, you care about her ... I care about her (more **for** her), but it is impossible for me to care about her as much as you do. Yes, I have 30 other patients in the ward, and yes, I have to worry about them the same as your mother, so I simply physically can't worry about your mother as much as you do. And also ... remember ... I have **my** mother to worry about ...

[5] A rural GP colleague's most recent complaint was that he had appeared 'dishevelled' at a home visit to a not particularly unwell patient ... at three in the morning.

[6] Hopefully obsolete by the time you read this book. A propaganda exercise where the Government pretends it has improved things by writing down all the things it would like to happen and saying they have happened, posting this up on hospital walls and telling the 'customer' to complain if they haven't.

2

Cardiology

The heart is dead easy.

If you ever actually meet a cardiologist, it shouldn't take long to realise that an abundance of neurons is no prerequisite for success in the specialty.[1] Admittedly this is partly because they have largely abandoned all semblance of clinical assessments, pinning their diagnostic decisions on the outcome of mod-tech investigations such as echocardiograms and exercise tolerance tests. A cardio-logical colleague of mine admitted recently he has used his stethoscope only once in the past three years, and that was at a medical conference in Buenos Aires to kill a tarantula. (It is a myth that the heavier heads of 'cardiology' stethoscopes are designed thus to reduce extraneous noise – the simple truth is that cardiologists are inclined to hold their conferences at the more exotic venues where the tarantulas tend to be bigger. The excessive price of the cardiology stethoscope exists so that the cardiologist will notice he's bought something. Cardiologists do rather well in the private sector.)

Cardiologists are, in fact, the physicians' equivalent of the consultant surgeon, right down to their pinstripe suits and shiny black shoes and even shinier big cars. While the outside world views surgeons as the only 'real' doctors in a hospital – leading them to consider anyone above the age of 35 who doesn't have a 'Mister'[2] in front of their name as some sort of failure – it does at least nod deferentially in the direction of the cardiologist as being a character of some import. This view is echoed in the media. The cardiologist's work is seen as more demanding – both intellectually and physically – than that of your standard punter physician. While many decades have passed since the Sports pages laboured under the mis-apprehension that big lumbering strikers were the heroes of the football world – having realised that centre-forwards scored more goals than other people because … like … er … they spent all their time lounging around the opponents' goal area – the surprisingly backward reaches of medical journalism seem fixed at the level of 'the heart – that's really important, isn't it? Those heart doctors must be

---

[1] That is, you don't need rocket science to realise you don't need rocket science to be a cardiologist.
[2] It has long troubled the more sensitive physicians that the general public believes all doctors become 'Mister' again after achieving a certain status. Many assume that any 'Doctor' cannot be a proper consultant. They are unaware that this is a change accorded specifically to surgeons upon attaining their Fellowship at one of the colleges. The explanation that traditionally surgeons were not doctors at all, but barbers, and that they did the cutting while doctors did the thinking (whether or not accompanied by any 'plus ca change' insinuations) is usually met by incredulous derision and is probably not worth pursuing. However, the knowledge of this is something to hold close to your physicianly heart to keep it warm on winter nights.

geniuses.' It is amazing how this clear fallacy can fool a surprising number of people, including those who should know better, notably the cardiologists themselves.

It is important for you, however, to be aware of the truth. If faced by the ostensibly daunting prospect of a cardiologist in an exam situation, then the advice of the other great guide in the English language – 'Don't Panic' – is of the essence. Keep things simple. Do not use any unnecessarily long words. Do not assume any major knowledge on the part of your ... opponent ... of any matters non-cardiological (and be careful not to overestimate their cardiology know-how). Be wary of trying to ingratiate yourself by attempting to engage their enthusiasm for outside interests. My own sortie in this direction, mentioning my brother-in-law's 27-foot yacht, was met by 'I didn't realise they still made them that size ...'

If these people can do it, so can you.

History

Cardiac history taking is simple – for reasons hinted at above. This is why cardiology outpatient appointments are usually over within ten minutes of the patient crossing the threshold (even allowing for one interruption on the consultant's mobile from his stockbroker). Basically it boils down to whether or not you have chest pain. If you do, you have an exercise tolerance test and maybe an angiogram. If not, an echocardiogram and maybe a 24-hour tape. Unless of course you see the cardiologist in a 'private' hospital, whereupon you automatically have all four tests organised – even if you're just the guy who's come in to fix the radiator.

Unfortunately, this approach is exclusively for the established cardiologist, and there is a requirement for some basic knowledge of symptomatology for the medical student and the junior doctor – respectively in order to pass exams or to assess and treat patients (a rather tedious duty which falls to the less well connected of the medical brotherhood). More happily, however, the knowledge itself is limited to two basic symptoms. Pain and breathlessness.

Pain

'Cardiac pain is tight ... heavy ... gripping ... the patient clenches his fist involuntarily when describing it (a dead giveaway) ... it radiates into the jaw ... and ... *particularly* ... the left arm ...'

All essentially true, but basically useless. Why? Because everybody knows all that. Everybody. That includes the patient. A generally unrecognised feature of the medical consultation, when we take a history in order to elicit a diagnosis, is that such diagnoses are made by knowing something about their symptoms that the patient doesn't. This isn't simply an exercise in one-upmanship. Once the patient has decided that they have, for example, angina, they will be delighted to give you the story that they know you want to hear. Thus you will only be making the diagnosis that the patient has already made for him- or herself – and what is the point of that? You might as well cut out the middle man and let them do their own coronary artery bypass graft (a study vetoed by a decidedly overzealous Ethics Committee in my last hospital). Symptoms lose their value once the patient knows about them. To my mind the best example of this is the 'pain going down the left arm' fallacy, and I present it thus:

> **Heresy Tip No. 1[3]**   **If a patient volunteers (i.e. before you have asked whether) that a chest pain goes into their left arm, then that pain is *less* likely to be cardiac.**

They've all read about it. They've all seen Superman's Dad having a heart attack consisting entirely of left arm pain (beautifully underplayed by Glen Ford). It's not that you can't trust patients (though we will be assessing this concept later). It's just that you can no longer trust the symptom. It has lost ... the element of surprise. Far be it from me to out-crazy the retired General in *Airplane* who refuses to put on the landing-lights to help the stricken passenger aircraft because '... that's exactly what they'll *expect* us to do ...', but I stand by the contention that the pain-going-right-down-the-left-arm pointer no longer points in the right direction.
   So.
   By all means ask the standard 'What was the pain like?' and 'Where did it go?' type questions, but always keep one eyebrow raised (this may be done either metaphorically or literally, depending on how much you wish to unsettle the patient). Better still, take the patient right through the whole story. Not only does this let the patient know you're a human being – not some interrogative automaton – but it also helps you to get a more genuine history. It also helps to build rapport with the patient. Ask what they were doing at the time (they will *always* say 'nothing', but persist and find out whether this nothing was standing, sitting watching TV, making the dinner, sitting eating, having sex with the neighbour's wife ...) and how the pain started – if it was sudden or 'crept up on them'. Ask if they felt absolutely OK except for the pain – 'I'm fine, but I got a pain' – or whether they had a feeling of just-not-being-a-well-person all of a sudden. The concept of a 'silent infarct' is well recognised in old people who may have no chest pain but simply a sudden breathlessness, faint or even 'not-wellness'. Yet we often ignore the importance of this not-wellness in younger people. They have the pain, but usually also get the not-wellness, and in its absence you have to at least consider other causes such as oesophageal pain. (Incidentally, oesophageal pain is an *outrageous* mimic of cardiac pain. Oesophageal spasm can feel the same, sound the same, respond to GTN and even cause T-wave inversion on the ECG tracing. Incidentally times two – patients will always say that the GTN took the pain away – even if they used their spray 30 seconds after the onset of a pain that went on to last 45 minutes. This will be described as 'my spray took it away eventually'.)
   This unwellness will often involve nausea, and may even go on to vomiting. Another well-known – and, despite this, probably correct – tenet is that ischaemic pain accompanied by vomiting is much more likely to be a myocardial infarction

---

[3] Occasionally the Cynical Tips will fly so much in the face of what is believed by every decent-living medical practitioner that they will be given the special status of Heresy Tips. The whole tip will be in bold type to make it especially easy **NOT TO READ IT.**

rather than simple angina (something to do with vagal tone, but this is hardly the place for such ... *medical* discussions). Experience suggests that this is true, though the caveat remains that this refers to pain already earmarked as *ischaemic* pain. The fact that a chest pain is accompanied by vomiting does not *per se* make it more likely that the pain is ischaemic in the first place.

This is a nice example of why 'history of presenting complaint' – going back in time to see how similar problems have affected the patient in the past – is of major help in diagnosing a current episode. If you've had angina in the past, it's more likely that the current episode is ischaemic in nature. Note, however, that this refers to 'having angina in the past', not 'saying you've had angina in the past'. This brings us rather abruptly to:

Heresy Tip No. 2   Don't believe a word the patient tells you.

I overstate. Both for effect and to give those who loom highest in my plans to have the book banned a useful sound bite. Closer to the truth is 'Don't assume that everything the patient tells you is correct'. They may say they have angina, but don't immediately write in your notes 'has angina'. No. Instead, ask 'Oh, how does it affect you?', and you will be amazed how often you are regaled with complaints which no more resemble angina than flying in the air.[4]

Stabbing pains probably isn't angina.

Breathlessness running for a bus probably isn't angina.

Pains-you-have-had-in-your-chest-for-the-past-27-years-which-come-on-at-any-time-of-day-no-matter-what-you-are-doing-including-nothing-at-all ... probably isn't angina.

All of the above hold true even if it has been 'diagnosed' as angina – whether by the patient's daughter who happens to be a nurse, the nextdoor neighbour who happens to have 'the same problem herself', or indeed the patient's GP who happens to be your best friend and who studied medicine alongside you for years and who certainly knew how to throw a ball in from the touchline, so you'd trust her with your life ...

And here, cautiously, we move on to ...

Cynical Tip No. 3[5]   Don't believe a word the patient's GP says.

Or, of course, 'don't assume that everything ... etc.'

Not only do GPs sometimes get things wrong – they are, after all, only human (and only just) – but also they are often obliged to come up with the diagnosis that most suits the patient. This might be for any of the financial, anti-stigmatic or

---

[4] As my mother would say, as in 'You're no more sick than flying in the air – get to school'.
[5] This started life as a Heresy Tip, but the concept is fast becoming so generally accepted that we may have to further downgrade it to a 'Don't Forget' Tip.

purely social reasons discussed earlier. Wear and tear from recurrent football trauma might be a more amenable diagnosis than the suggestion that obesity is the main culprit. Indeed, arriving at the same diagnosis as the patient, her nursing daughter or her identically affected neighbour is often the only way for the GP to avoid a long protracted dispute as to whether his diagnostic skills honed in some posh university can possibly stand up against the superior approach of the University of Life enthusiast who 'should know my own body' or indeed that of their next door neighbour. It is a well-established fact in the letters pages of newspapers at all levels that a doctor who holds out against the diagnostic decisions of a layperson is in need of being taken down a peg or two. Better therefore on many occasions for the GP to fall in with the patient's wishes and attach some hopefully harmless label to their complaints.

So.

Don't accept 'angina' as a past diagnosis. Get the story. Find out whether the pain[6] does indeed come on with exercise and resolve within a few minutes of resting. This is probably more important than the site of the pain, which can crop up in the most bizarre of places. I've seen patients whose well-documented angina is always in the abdomen, or the side of the face. This can confuse the attending physician when they turn up at Casualty. And this leads us nicely into another important principle.

Never decide that what the patient describes as angina definitely isn't. Just because it doesn't fit your, my, or anyone else's preconceived notions doesn't exclude this or any other condition. When we refuse to assume that the patient or their GP has the correct diagnosis, we should never replace this with the assumption that we *do* have. Things change. Things surprise us. We are always learning (and, of course, increasingly after the age of 30, forgetting). Keep an open mind – that's the secret.

> **Cynical Tip No. 4** (borrowed from local cardiologist) When seeing a patient in clinic, if they rub their chest with a slightly rotatory motion, saying '... I've got it just now ...', this isn't angina.

Where were we?

Oh yeah. Acute chest pain. One intriguing feature of chest pain is the duration. As the minutes move up towards 30 it becomes less likely that the pain is simple angina and more likely that it is a myocardial infarction. MI remains the more likely until about two hours, after which its likelihood recedes and paradoxically angina becomes the better bet (the old-fashioned 'unstable' angina of 'acute coronary syndrome', which can of course lead on to an infarct at some stage in its evolution) – or an entirely non-ischaemic alternative. This doesn't mean that the patient *can't* have an infarct at some stage during the prolonged pain, but the pain following a short sharp MI is rarely prolonged. The pain itself is so variable we find ourselves relying more and more on ...

---

[6] Indeed, note whether they call it 'pain'. Patients with proper angina often dismiss 'pain' as a suitable word for their discomfort.

Accompanying symptoms

It's nice if a patient can mention these voluntarily. It's rarely convincing if you ask concerning dizziness, breathlessness, sweating and nausea to be met with a slight pause followed by 'yes' to every question. I am always more convinced if the patient can muster a 'no' to at least one. Alternatively, one could (as suggested by an ex-colleague who now works in Inverness[7] − if that tells you anything) toss in what the Americans might term a 'curve-ball', the English a 'googly' and presumably the Invernesshireans a 'caber from off-field'. Ask if the patient has, say, haemoptysis. (I am, of course, suggesting you ask about 'coughing up blood' − though on further reflection an answer of 'yes' to 'have you any haemoptysis?' might well give you the information you seek.) An answer in the negative will help to reinforce the veracity of the patient's other complaints.

With regard to 'sweating', I always ask patients if it was a 'hot' or 'cold' sweat. With absolutely no good evidence to back up my case (the more perspicacious reader will be noting a recurring theme), I have come to the conclusion that a *cold* sweat is more indicative of a severe episode of ischaemic pain. Again, this may be some autonomic … vagal … pain severity thing (hot sweats happen when you're hot and need to lose heat − or if your hypothalamus is fooled into believing this − and cold sweats are an autonomic reaction to pain/fear, etc.), but I really cannot afford to get bogged down by medical facts in a treatise such as this which depends entirely on personal prejudices.

Breathlessness

The only other symptom in the cardiovascular household worth a moment of your time is breathlessness. Here, one single factor is more important to your future success than any other. You have to decide how best to pronounce 'dyspnoea'. This is crucial. You must find a pronunciation which is appropriate to your station, but lets others know that you are … a contender. To my mind, 'diss-knee-a' [dis‚ni'a], with the accent on the 'knee', is the 'normal' pronunciation. As far as I can remember, when I was a student, *everybody* pronounced it like that. Part of this may have been a regional effect, since my entire medical childhood was spent in the West of Scotland where, for example, no one puts an 'r' in the middle of 'drawing' or at the end of 'law'.[8] However, leaving aside the influence of incomers who think 'tis better to give received pronunciation, I believe that specialties breed their own pronunciations − a way of showing you are above the standard punter, a shibboleth[9] which lets others know we have one of the cognoscenti[10] here. Optional pronunciations have thus evolved. 'Diss-ny-a' [dis'nia‚] with the stress on the 'diss' − is the real alternative, with the two other options formed by electing

---

[7] A big town in the Scottish Highlands − hugely north of Watford and just short of *ultima Thule*.

[8] Our only excuse − though a very good one − is that … well, there isn't any 'r' in either of these positions and there is no reason why one should pretend that there is. Also, as the people of Scotland are actually able to pronounce 'r's properly (or 'roll them', as some would have it), the superfluous sound becomes quite intrusive.

[9] Shibboleth: catchword by which members of a group may be recognised. From biblical times when the ability to pronounce 'sh' could help to distinguish one tribe from another. Now the word itself is used by writers who would like themselves to be taken seriously as a member of the writing fraternity.

[10] See last sentence of last footnote.

to pronounce the hitherto 'silent p' ('as in bath' as they say at faux-risqué dinner parties) giving us 'diss-p-nee-a' [dis͵pni'a] and 'diss-pnia' [dis'pnia,][11]. One would have thought that consulting a good dictionary would help us to resolve the issue, but unfortunately this is not the case. While some are quite explicit on the subject ... none of them quite agrees with me.

Despite this, I stand by the stance (physiologically interesting) that diss-knee-a is the standard student and ordinary doctor pronunciation. However, if you wish to be thought of as one of the 'cardiology boys' (or girls, but you will have gleaned from the general picture of cardiologists that this is not a burgeoning group), then you should make a point of adopting whichever of the three options outlined above is the flavour of the month – usually the flavour of the local professor.

Fortunately, this dilemma does not encroach upon our history taking from the patient, since you will not be using the word 'dyspnoea' in this situation – unless they happen to be a medical practitioner, in which case it is your duty to immediately down tools (even those for splitting infinitives) and go fetch someone much more senior who is more likely to ask all the right questions, despite never having been asked to do so for the last six years.

It is difficult to get a grasp of dyspnoea. Some define it as simply 'an awareness of breathing', since normally we aren't. But that seems plain silly. Not only would it include a multitude of psychogenic scenarios – indeed 'awareness of breathing' *per se* would seem to me a more psychogenic description than anything else – but we'd clearly have to view James Bond, hiding in hopeful silence in the Underground Installation meeting-room's cupboard, as being 'dyspnoeic'. No. To keep the term at all useful, we have to keep it fairly synonymous with 'breathless'. But then, what is *breathless*? Patients often find it difficult to differentiate breathlessness from fatigue (e.g. on walking). I've tried – in a flash of inspiration – asking if they feel after walking, say, 50 yards as if they'd run the 50 yards or if they had walked 5 miles – but it didn't appear to help.

Dyspnoea at rest they usually find easier to differentiate. We often ask patients if their dyspnoea is worse in any particular position (e.g. lying down). This 'orthopnoea' (and here I find myself oddly happy to pronounce the 'p' ... my stance on the subject is becoming less and less tenable) has been largely hijacked by the cardiologists as a major pointer towards pulmonary oedema ... left ventricular failure ... 'cardiac' dyspnoea. But to be honest, *most* dyspnoeas are worse when lying flat. Asthma certainly is. That funny coughing/breathless thing you get with a virus in winter (maybe a mild version of asthma itself) seems to be. And any time you watch some athlete finish a marathon or the 10 000 metres and lie flat on the ground, they're pretty quick to get themselves up again and continue their recovery in at least a seated position.

So pretty much any dyspnoea is worse when lying down. Maybe that qualification simply helps to define it as dyspnoea, and not one of those fatigue things I was all worried about. The breathlessness which occasionally wakes you up (paroxysmal nocturnal dyspnoea – PND) might be a more specific pointer to cardiac causes (though not entirely specific), but is probably more useful for

---

[11] Interestingly, the main ophthalmology shibboleth concerns the pronunciation of exclusive wines such as *Le Montrachet*. Here, the received wisdom is to follow the classic French and omit to pronounce the 't'. It is to be noted that this refers to the central 't'. Any of you who were even thinking about pronouncing the terminal 't' should seriously consider a career as an orthopaedic surgeon.

showing up the practitioner's true origins – since most of the dis-p-nya acolytes will resort to 'normal' pronunciation when using the phrase 'paroxysmal nocturnal dyspnoea' (listen out – you'll hear what I mean).

To be honest, dyspnoea is a rather dull symptom compared with the excitement of its pronunciation. It's tricky to tell one cause from another. The only worthwhile feature is probably how bad it is and if it's getting worse. Even that can be difficult to elucidate from most patients, since it is almost unheard of to see one whose dyspnoea is gradually getting better.

Palpitation(s)

OK. I said there were only two cardiac symptoms, but I suppose we must mention palpitations. Again, the word itself is much more exciting than the symptom. First, does it have an 's'? Technically, a burst of 300 heart beats in 60 seconds is a palpitation (assuming the patient has spotted it – but we'll get to that), but the patient will almost certainly call it 'palpitations' – i.e. each beat is a palpitation. The nicety rarely causes trouble, since most patients will have had more than one episode, so everyone can happily talk about the *palpitations* (unless the patient wishes them to be *palpitationses*). The definition is also similar to dyspnoea – 'abnormal awareness of the heart beat'. It doesn't have to be in the chest and it doesn't have to be fast. The heart 'missing a beat' is a palpitation, usually caused by an extrasystole, and the patient is also aware of the subsequent compensatory pause. They are rarely of any significance. To be honest, most palpitations are rarely of any significance – but that's only *most* of them ... so find out what they're like and when the patient gets them.

For years I've asked patients to tap out their palpitation – hoping to discover without witness-leading whether they are regular or irregular, and indeed how fast they are – to no avail. Whether they are able to recite 40 bars from *La Bohème* or Eminem, all patients are singularly unable to give any rendition of this episode which causes so much concern. Even giving them an option between

      Rat ... tat ... tat ... tat ... tat ... tat ... tat ... tat ...

and

      Rat ... tat ...... tat . tat ... tat . tat .. tat . tat ...... tat .. tat
      ... tat . tat . tat ...... tat ...

will simply result in their choosing the second one no matter which order you do them in. (Or echo Kevin Klein in *A Fish Called Wanda* by asking 'What was the middle one again?')

After failing to elicit the rhythm, it's easy to find oneself 'on a roll' and equally fail to identify any precipitant factors such as stress, coffee, coca-cola or cigarettes,[12] or any post-hoc pointers such as abrupt polyuria (an association with

---

[12] It comes as a perennial surprise to smokers that nicotine is a stimulant (both neurological and cardiac – hence its relevance here). They are seduced by the idea that a cigarette 'relaxes them', stubbornly oblivious of the fact that it can only do this by relieving their withdrawal symptoms once they are hooked. The reason so many smokers can reduce their intake to exactly four per day is probably less to do with mealtimes than with the half-life of nicotine, although the two may be related, as eating increases nicotine breakdown.

paroxysmal supraventricular tachycardia I've espoused for many years with nary a hit to back it up). While accompanying features such as chest pain and dizziness may give some indication of the haemodynamic 'seriousness' of any dysrhythmia, one helpful feature is how the palpitation *ended*. A stress-induced or other sinus tachycardia is likely to end gradually, while SVTs, AF and indeed VT (one way or the other) are more likely to end abruptly.

Awareness of the sound of the heart beating or of the pulse in an artery while lying in bed is not a significant palpitation, and suggests that the sufferer hasn't enough other things to worry about in bed at night.

Oedema

All right, four. It gets worse as the day goes on, just so you can tell it's not arthritis.

Examination

It is worth spending time on examination of the cardiovascular system. It will *always* be in *any* medical exam. You might easily go through an entire medical career and never examine cranial nerves under exam conditions[13] – perhaps never an abdomen – but there will always be a heart, or at the very least a pulse.

There are two reasons for this. First, the heart is (arguably) quite important. Secondly, every physician in the world thinks they are good at it. So the guy examining you examining the heart thinks he knows what he is doing, even if earlier he couldn't decide which side of the chest the damn thing was in when auscultating the patient himself. All clinical examinations of any importance are now preceded by an allocated period for the examiners to examine (we will *have* to do something about this double meaning for 'examine') the patients who have agreed to help (or 'clinical material', as those of you who have opted for the 'diss-p-nya' approach should by now be calling them). Ostensibly this is to give the examiners the chance to check that the information on their crib-sheets is correct. The real function is to let the registrar who has organised the exam show the examiners how to elicit the various clinical signs which would otherwise elude their atrophied skills.[14] Thus does an Interlocutor at the College Exams fail a candidate for examining for mitral stenosis in precisely the same manner as the Interlocutor himself had used 30 minutes earlier. All he needed was a little reminder to restore him to his normal status of expert cardiac-examiner-examiner.

You see, everybody thinks that the heart is important (I blame Shakespeare), so everybody who wants to take themselves at all seriously as a doctor likes to think that they can 'do the heart'. Thus, while you might get away with major blunders in examining, say, the musculoskeletal system (after all, who gives a monkey's? It won't kill them, it'll still be sore tomorrow – and somebody else who's interested in that sort of thing can have a look), the slightest slip in

---

[13] If fastidiously careful at bedside teaching sessions, you might never examine them at all.

[14] It is a moot point whether skills of no great moment in the first place can atrophy. Since the phrase 'cerebral atrophy' is used with general abandon, however …

examining the heart can be fatal career-wise. They think that you *should* be able to do it, because they *can*.

Numerous books deal with clinical examination of the CVS better than I can hope to – mainly because they are written by people who have themselves read a book – so we must confine ourselves to one or two basic tips as we go to 'examine the cardiovascular system'.

It is always at this stage that the student asks 'Should I tell you about it as I go along or do you want me to wait till the end?' This question is, of course, only of relevance when it comes to exams (though the regimentation of some is taking away any option). My advice is to do, without asking, whichever way you feel you are best at (or most comfortable with, if you can't tell). If the examiner doesn't care, you get to do it the way you want. If the examiner prefers your way, they will be pleased that you like the same way. If they prefer the other way, they will tell you politely and you can change. Do not worry. They will not hold it against you, and might even view your performance extra favourably in the light of your doing it in an unaccustomed fashion. Any which way, you win.

General

Examination for anaemia is generally considered to be part of cardiological examination. The best place is the conjunctivae – pulling down the lower lid with the tip of your thumb to see whether these look normal or deathly pale. Note that the thumb is used, rather than a poking index finger. Much less momentarily distressing for the patient. Honest! Try it yourself with your own eye. See? Depending on your personal preference, move smoothly on to either hands or pulse

Pulse

Do feel lots of them. Get used to normal (and abnormal) pulses so that you don't start making up nonsense when it comes to an exam. If you've only felt five pulses in five years (and one belonged to a female colleague at an end-of-term party when you were just making sure ...) then you're going to struggle to decide whether a pulse volume is normal or not. ('actually ... I can hardly hear it at all ... maybe it should be turned up ...').

Do feel the pulses in both arms – but don't take forever over it. This is true of lots of things you 'have to do' under examination conditions in medicine. It's like looking in the mirror during the driving test. You've *got* to do it, and the examiner's got to see you doing it, but you don't pass by showing off a long and lingering look in the rear-view mirror while smacking into a lamp-post. So you check the pulse, make sure it's the same as the other one, then leave it. Don't double your time to take the pulse – leaving less time to show off your extensive knowledge and interpretive powers. (*Never* think it is a good idea to take an inordinately long time to do a simple examination, hoping that this will use up the time which you might otherwise spend squirming under awkward questions. First, examiners aren't daft. Secondly, examiners are very easily irritated.)

Do study the crest for the Royal College of Physicians of London for a view of an Omnipotent Being's hand coming down from above to take the pulse of a disembodied arm. *Do not*, however, copy its technique, as only Omnipotent Beings can consistently feel pulses on the *ulnar* side of the wrist.

Do follow the age-old system – **R**ate, **R**hythm, **V**olume, **C**haracter, **C**ondition of **V**essel **W**all (easily remembered by the catchy mnemonic RRVCCVW) – but don't emphasise that you are following it. Thus 'The pulse is 80 per minute, regular with normal volume ...', not 'The rate is 80 beats per minute, the rhythm is regular, the ... er ... character ... no, sorry, the ... er ... volume is ...'

The added benefit of avoiding the 'ticking-off-a-list' presentation (as well as the more pleasing fluidity of the answer) is that if you do miss something out, the examiner will probably not notice (unless it is very important, e.g. the only positive finding in the whole case – in which case 'Hell mend you', as my mother would say.[15] This book ain't out to help people pass exams who shouldn't be allowed to pass exams.[16] Actually, now I remember, this book ain't out to help people pass exams).

Rate is expressed in beats per minute – though you don't have to say 'beats'. Nor, when writing it down, is it necessary to give the simple test some ersatz scientific legitimacy by stating it as '80 min^{-1}'. Take it over 15 seconds and multiply by ... four. Statistically speaking, you will get a more representative figure by counting over half an hour and dividing by 30, but this method is not advised (even if your need to avoid awkward questions borders on the pathological). Perhaps this would be an appropriate place to introduce the most traditional of tips.

Betting Tip No. 1   Unscrupulous money can be won from physicians of any level by betting them that they cannot define both bradycardia and tachycardia. While trying to avoid the question by making trite complaints that it depends on the situation, most will eventually make a guess, since it clearly seems the sort of thing they should know. The true definitions are that tachycardia is 100 beats/minute and above (i.e. 100 beats/minute is a tachycardia) and that bradycardia is below 60 beats/minute (i.e. 60 beats/minute is normal and bradycardia starts at 59 beats/minute). Almost no one will get both right.[17]

Rhythm is 'regular' or 'irregular' or 'regular with ...' 'Sinus rhythm' is a description that can only be made on seeing an ECG tracing (in a similar vein, when shown an ECG tracing, it would not be sufficient to describe the rhythm as regular). The phrase 'irregularly irregular' is a clear bit-of-fun-Dougal which has apparently caught the imagination of medical practitioners for centuries. Much loved by everyone, despite being obvious nonsense, I can only advise that you stick with it

---

[15] As in 'If you think flying in the air is a good idea, then Hell mend you'.
[16] An interesting 'ethical' dilemma: many of the things we teach students aren't really to help examine patients, or look after them better, but to help students pass exams. If you had a student (at undergraduate or postgraduate level) who you really felt should *not* pass the exam, as they might be a danger to the public ... and you had this really neat trick that impressed in exams ... should you ... tell it to them? Should you teach them any 'examination technique' at all?
[17] More money can be made by provoking a bet that Edinburgh is not west of Liverpool, but it may be difficult to drop this into the conversation without arousing suspicion.

as the description of the random pulse associated with atrial fibrillation (AF). Remember that there is no such thing as fast or slow AF, since the fibrillation is always pretty much the same, but the *ventricular response* is variable. Cardiologists occasionally like to be precise about this (though the reasons are unclear, since it is unlikely to alter their invoices in any way). Asking students for 23 causes of atrial fibrillation and similar questions is now thoroughly frowned upon. Such questions will, however, still be asked by some sad examiners – like myself – who adore such things, if only because of their very being-frowned-uponicity. The answer is 'ischaemic heart disease, rheumatic heart disease – in particular mitral stenosis, thyrotoxicosis, hypert–', at which point the examiner will stop you.[18] The secret is to start as if you will indeed recite all 23 causes.

Volume can be large, normal or small. Alternatively it may be high, normal or low. Do not use descriptions such as 'good' (Is that larger than normal?) or 'thready' (What exactly would a thready volume be? A 1929 copy of Proust's *De Cote de Chez Swan* with the cover falling off?). The pulse volume in atrial fibrillation just has to be variable. Presumably this means that different examiners with different sensitivities in their fingertips will actually count different numbers of beats when trying to calculate the pulse rate in AF. This is reason enough to emphasise that the 'pulse deficit' – that popular difference between the perceived heart rate measured at the wrist and the actual ventricular rate – is of no numerical significance. A pulse deficit of 20 is no 'worse' than one of 10. Its only significance indeed is to remind you that the ventricular rate *will* be different from that measured at the wrist – and the ventricular rate is what counts. Rapid ventricular rate with poor LV output may produce a 'normal' rate at the wrist.

Character. Please consult a *proper* medical textbook – though the famous collapsing pulse is worth a mention. This is something you are required to test for specifically in exams even if the pulse character doesn't suggest for a moment that it might be even thinking about collapsing. The collapsing pulse usually goes up very quickly, and certainly falls precipitously. This makes sense when you think of the main cause – aortic incompetence, where the blood immediately starts to flow backwards through the leaky valve as soon as it shuts. The classic check is, with the patient's arm slightly raised, to attempt to feel the pulse at the patient's wrist (for budding surgeons, this is on the *palmar* side) using the upper palm of your own hand at about your metacarpo-phalangeal joint level. Cardiology cognoscenti often try this further up the patient's arm – though attempts to show off with this manoeuvre are likely to meet with unimpressed bewilderment in the uninitiated examiner. The theory is that a normal pulse isn't usually palpable like this, but a collapsing one often is. Not the best test, really. It's one of those attempts to quantify something which is essentially a subjective finding of a fast-dropping large-volume pulse which experience will identify when taking the pulse at the wrist. Trying to put some yes/no quantitative test to it – like deciding whether turquoise is blue or green.[19] Again the real secret goes back to my first point on examining the pulse. The more of them you actually feel, the more likely you are to spot when there is a collapsing pulse – or some other abnormality – and not fall back on some test that you've only been encouraged to do in patients who

---

[18] In case the examiner is late with his line, the next bit is '-ension'.
[19] Measuring the blood pressure is reputed to settle any difficult instances – the collapsing pulse having a large pulse pressure (systolic minus diastolic). Unfortunately, no one knows how large that

had a collapsing pulse! The bottom line is not to go back on your feeling that a pulse might be collapsing just because some bizarre test doesn't come up with the goods.

Collapsing pulses are so ingrained in the medical exam psyche that even in their absence you might be asked for causes. The trap here is to rhyme off all the causes of a simple large-volume ('bounding') pulse. Fever, pregnancy, anaemia and thyrotoxicosis do *not* cause a collapsing pulse. Its specific fast-up fast-down character can only be caused by three things – aortic incompetence, patent ductus arteriosus (PDA) and arterio-venous shunts – of which the first is by far the most commonly presented to you.

Now. There is a need for shrewdness here. Not everybody knows the above, including not every examiner. So when they ask for all the causes, they often *do* want you to rhyme off all of the wrong answers as outlined. Here we for the first time encounter the rules of engagement for examinations.

Examination Rule No. 1 Never argue with the examiner.

Unfortunately, Rule somewhere-in-the-middle-of-the-teens for Life (among those of us who like to hold on to some smidgeon of integrity and self-respect) is *never agree with something you know not to be true*. To be fair, this is a rule which many – not just in the medical profession – find impossible not to jettison at some point along the way. However, I personally believe that it is worth holding on to for as long as you can, though this is not the route to rapid advancement. In the present case, luckily, there is a way out. The answer is to pre-empt the examiner's response if you suspect the above calamity is about to occur – for instance, if he has previously asked for 23 causes of atrial fibrillation. You therefore say 'Causes are aortic regurgitation, patent ductus arteriosus and arterio-venous shunts ...' followed quickly, allowingnotimeforinterruption, by 'You can also get a "bounding" pulse with fever, pregnancy, anaemia and thyrotoxicosis – though these are not true collapsing pulses'.

An old boss of mine once told me he only gave a pass mark in the Membership exam to a candidate who had taught him something.[20] It is best to fulfil this requirement without the rest of the world realising.

---

would have to be. Large pulse pressures may occur with the bounding pulses mentioned above – while blood pressure measurement is shamelessly inaccurate in any case. Most people write down a blood pressure which makes sense, rather than what they have actually measured. Using classical techniques, the pulse sound often refuses to go away as you gradually release the cuff (rendering any Korotkoff$_5$ measurement as zero), while any attempt to define when these muffled sounds become ... more ... muffled (K$_4$) is optimistic in the extreme. It is an enlightening experience to compare a 'new page' of a patient's blood pressure recordings with the previous one. Having varied slightly around one focal blood pressure for the entire previous week, the patient's blood pressure will magically find a new fulcrum as a nurse puts down a genuine reading to start the new page. Subsequent nurses then adapt their measurements to conform towards this new norm.

[20] This same old boss had a very 'psychological' approach to his patients (though I often suspected that his need for me to come down from the ward to take blood was more to do with laziness than the declared avoidance of a disruption to the psychological rapport he was building). His probing included asking patients how they would like to meet their death (no threat intended) – his own stated preference being to die at the age of 87, having been shot by a jealous husband.

> **Examination Rule No. 2** Never embarrass the examiner (or, as a rider to Rule No.1, if you do find you are arguing with the examiner, then make sure that you don't win).

Students don't realise that the pressure in an examination goes both ways. It is actually quite taxing and intimidating to be examining students or postgraduates. This is usually exacerbated by examining in pairs, where you have a colleague whom you wouldn't necessarily wish to impress, but who you certainly don't want to have watching while you make a fool of yourself. Many years ago a trainee colleague of mine found himself thrust into the role of Finals Examiner, paired with the 'External' while still himself a Senior Registrar. Running out of questions to ask in an open-ended viva (as you do!), he asked the distinction student (now a national figure in cardiology) about the prophylaxis of malaria. He relaxed back as the student impressed him with chat on erythrocytic and exo-erythrocytic phases which all seemed eminently sensible. Eventually the 'External' said that he felt he 'had to intervene', revealed himself to be a Professor of Tropical Medicine at a forefront Tropical Medicine Department which specialised in ... (you'll have guessed), and pointed out that the student had been talking the most 'unadulterated balderdash' for the past five minutes 'and Doctor X has just been letting you!'

So don't forget to give the examiners a break once in a while. They're under pressure, too.

The other pulse character worth mentioning is the slow-rising and slow-falling 'plateau pulse'. Its association with aortic stenosis makes so much sense that no more needs to be said.

State of the vessel wall. Who cares?

Hands

Another quandary. You're looking at a normal pair of hands. Do you say they're normal, or do you start spieling off all the things that are not there?

There is no easy answer to this. A lot depends on your style — and that of the examiner. It would be embarrassing to say that the hands are normal, and then find the grossly abnormal bits (or, worse, have them pointed out to you ... '... and how many fingers does one normally find on, say, the left hand?'). On the other hand (... leave it), you don't want to bore the examiner with a big long list of things which aren't there ('*no* clubbing, *no* splinter haemorrhages, *no* sixth finger ...'). If you fill in the sort of time you'd normally take to look at the hands, while mentioning the major negatives (a nice touch here is to point out a negative when the clinical history or earlier examination might suggest that it will be present), that should work out about right. It shows your systematic approach, gives you a verbal reminder about what you're doing, but doesn't go on too long.

If you're examining the hands in relation to a specific system ('this man has a problem with his heart — could you examine the hands please?'), then confining yourself to negatives (and to some extent positives) which relate to that system makes sense. ('Very interesting, Mr Smith. What rheumatological causes of leuconychia were you thinking of?'). In the same vein, if you are examining the hands in, for example, a cardiological mode and mention clubbing, then you should meet any request for causes with the cardiological causes first. Indeed the examiner should pursue things no further once you have confidently mentioned infective endocarditis[21] and cyanotic congenital heart disease – except to ask for at least one example of the latter to show that you have the slightest clue what you are talking about. Probably the best choice here is any Eisenmenger's syndrome (where an initially left-to-right shunt becomes right-to-left[22]), both because of the ease with which one can explain the cyanosis, and the fact that all clinicians just love the word 'Eisenmenger's' – with good reason. Say it aloud. Now (unless you are on a bus, in which case you shouldn't really be reading as you'll make yourself sick). It's a brilliant word. **Eisenmenger's**. Great.

Anaemia may be legitimately looked for in the creases of the palm of the hand. It would be optimistic to hazard any guess at actual haemoglobin levels – though I occasionally insist that a student does so, if only to emphasise Examination Rule No. 1. Using the creases to forecast the patient's longevity or whether they will marry a lawyer and have three children is a definite no-no, even among those who refuse to dismiss reflexology and other suchness as the entirely-unbased-on-anything-sensible pieces of chicanery that they may well be (*see* Chapter 8 on alternative medicine).

Koilonychia (flattening – going on to 'spooning' of the nails) is also a legitimate sign – of iron deficiency. Not to be confused with being a sign of anaemia, since a transfusion of six units of blood will not instantly change the shape of your nails.

Splinter haemorrhages are small, thin, almost brown marks (if you're Scottish, it'll help if I tell you that they look like a skelf) in the nail near the hyponychium (that's the bit where the muck collects) running longitudinally (i.e. not across the nail) – and can occur in infective endocarditis or in vasculitic diseases such as systemic lupus erythematosus (SLE).[23] Their frequency is perhaps summed up by my own reaction to seeing them recently in a patient. Twenty thousand years' experience in rheumatology enabled me to comment 'what on earth is that?' (or words to that effect).

Clubbing is a pain in the neck. Not only does no one have any idea what causes it, but any attempt to verify its existence leads to unsurmountable

---

[21] It is one of those annoying foibles of modern nomenclature that you will almost certainly be corrected if you say 'subacute bacterial endocarditis' in this situation, as this term has been supplanted by 'infective endocarditis'. This despite the unlikelihood of any form of infective endocarditis (essentially an umbrella term) other than the subacute variety having time to cause clubbing.

[22] For example, a significant ventricular septal defect (VSD) where the right ventricle has to deal with the excess blood leaking into it (from the left) during systole. This extra work leads to hypertrophy and increased pressure in the RV until it becomes greater than that in the LV and the shunt is reversed – so 'blue' unoxygenated blood goes direct from the RV into the LV and into the arterial system. *Seems* to make sense. But ... now that the LV is getting extra blood ... will it hypertrophy and reverse the flow back to normal? Or, to put it another way, how does the RV pressure actually get *above* that of the left (probably all complicated by changes in the pulmonary vasculature)? Or, indeed, what happens when the pressures are equal? Are you (briefly) cured?

[23] SLE always fascinated me as a student. Its name kept cropping up as the cause of things – indeed became the stock guess when one hadn't a clue – without my ever getting an idea what it actually was. Like Godot. Today, after said 20 years in rheumatology, I feel no closer to any real understanding. Ah well, nothing to be done.

difficulties. The 'clubbing' we all immediately spot is essentially the beaking of the nail – an increase in its longitudinal curvature – that is often but not always associated with clubbing itself. So somebody, somewhere, comes up with a precise definition. 'Loss of the nail-angle.' Which always left me with a problem. What nail-angle? Between what and ... what? I remember nodding sagely when first told about this during bedside teaching, but my life experience, anatomy lessons ... even guitar lessons had never introduced me to the concept of my having some nail-angle that I might later make use of. Out of fear of appearing stupid in front of my student peers, I said nothing – only to find later that no one else knew what the tutor had been talking about.

Even now I remain uncertain, but it appears that if you look across the top of your finger, from the side, there is an obtuse angle as the skin/cuticle dips down towards the nail and then the nail itself moves up at a slight angle. But, I hear you cry, every one of my nails looks slightly different ... and in some of them there's almost no angle there ...

Precisely.

Anyways. Apparently clubbing is the filling in of this nail-angle so that the nail seems to go straight on from the skin. One way to demonstrate this is to put the distal phalanges of two opposing fingers nail to nail. Normally this will give you a kite-shaped (admittedly a very thin kite, which could no more waft exuberantly in a Force 4 breeze than would a size-14 knitting needle) space between the fingers. With clubbing this disappears (Patrick's test). At this point I usually point out the obvious, that it also disappears if you've got fat fingers, but ... it doesn't. Patrick's test may actually work (if indeed it is Patrick's test. My memory's not what it was. That might be the test for whether the chicken's ready[24]). Certainly better than all that extra fluctuance in the nail bed nonsense that we like to use to back up the story. All base-of-nail beds are fluctuant to some degree, again with major inter-patient (and intra-patient[25]) variation.

Personally, I feel that no one has ever diagnosed an illness on the basis of the fingers being clubbed, so all the 'Do you think the fingers are clubbed?' conversations serve no purpose. You have to view any sign with some suspicion when the most likely cause is 'idiopathic'. Most fingers are diagnosed as clubbed after an associated-with-finger-clubbing diagnosis has been established and retro-spectively someone can look at the hands and say 'Aha! That's why the fingers are clubbed'.

Cyanosis could be considered as cardiological or respiratory. Since the former specialty already has an over-inflated view of its importance, let's leave it to the respiratory section. That way I also save one of my favourite trick questions for later, whilst allowing myself some *schadenfreude* in annoying any reader keen to learn cyanosis's secrets. Presumably the same emotion felt by those appendix compilers who spurn my efforts in negotiating the alphabet, rewarding me with a 'see elsewhere'. As in 'PSS – *see* Progressive Systemic Sclerosis' so we find 'Progressive Systemic Sclerosis – *see* Systemic Sclerosis' whereupon 'Systemic

---

[24] You stick a size-14 knitting needle into the flesh and see if the juice runs clear. Don't use a kite (or indeed a peregrine falcon – they're illegal and don't taste as good).

[25] *Inter* – difference between one patient and another. *Intra* – difference within the one patient. Other medical use is the inter-observer variation (different observer) vs. intra-observer (same observer, different occasion) in statistics and research. If confused, think *international* football match.

Sclerosis' reveals 'see Scleroderma', which when found exhorts me to 'see PSS' (OK, it actually says 'P 546', but my point is that it would be much easier for everybody if they all said that). This may be an alternative explanation to the obvious one as to why, in my hospital library's copy of *Bailey and Love's Short*[26] *Practice of Surgery*, the appendix has been removed.

The most difficult item in the entire examination of the entire body

Before moving from the hands to the precordium, we are paradoxically allowed just a few seconds to deal with the most difficult item in the entire examination of the entire body ... entirely.

Jugular venous pulse (JVP)

This is it. The hardest thing there is. The examination that even the most experienced of physicians will nine times out of ten simply pretend to do. But you are expected to do it right − under exam conditions!

In my opinion, every teacher you get in your undergraduate years can teach you three, maybe four things that are worthwhile. Everybody's got these genuine little nuggets that they've picked up along the way. They themselves may not even recognise them. Yet, whether it be subliminal or otherwise, they'll manage to manoeuvre their first sessions so that these pearls of wisdom will be scattered in your trough of despond by the time you have moved on to your next guru and his or her own sparkling gems. Now I believe (with no certainty) that one of my juiciest nuggets (alongside 'better a mixed metaphor than a ludicrously extended one') concerns the JVP. So, early in our relationship, I always ask my students ...

'What colour is the JVP?'

Some simply look perplexed. Some − revealing themselves as the ones requiring enlightenment − suggest 'blue'. Only the very occasional hero replies 'skin-coloured'.

One sure-fire way to fail in your quest for the JVP is to look for a blue column of blood. It's the *internal jugular vein* which you seek, the one everybody emphasises is between the heads of sterno-cleido-mastoid, but doesn't mention that while the unhelpful *external jugular* which lies lateral to this is usually blue ... the *internal* pulse is well under the surface and is seen as a wobbling of normal-coloured skin.

The positioning of the patient at 45° is, of course, an entirely arbitrary figure that gives you a fair chance of seeing the pulse in position. What are the chances that any genuine alignment of the root of the superior vena cava and the angle of Louis (the flange where the manubrium meets the sternum proper and whence all good students measure their JVPs) will occur at exactly half of a right-angle?[27] If it were all so precise, then the 'normal' level which is allowable wouldn't vary

---

[26] It is unclear whether the 'short' suggests they encourage doing operations very quickly or whether 'short practice' suggests a brief career. Maybe both.

[27] The theory being that in this position the angle of Louis is always 5 cm above the mid-right atrium, so the actual jugular venous pressure is what we measure plus 5 cm.

from 2 to 5 centimetres (is it anything more than coincidence that 2 inches = 5 centimetres? I only ask because the normal chest expansion is also defined as 5 centimetres (2 inches), while we only start to take decreased chest expansion seriously at the 2 cm level. Does this all come from some vague mix-up in the collective mind of medics? Or do things really start to bother you when they are outwith (shouldn't really use that word, as apparently it doesn't exist outwith Scotland) the normal by a ratio of 2.54:1?) depending on which textbook you read.[28]

However, it remains a harmless convention that one ignores at one's peril. So get the patient (gently) to lie at approximately 45°, but don't spend a protractored amount of time doing it. Get them to gently turn their unstretched head slightly to the left, and look for their right JVP pulse between those infamous heads of sterno-cleido-mastoid. Change your angle of vision a couple of times (look at opposite side), as it can be easier to see side-on. It's just a wobble of skin. Classically a double-pulse — **a**(trial contraction) and **v**(enous filling) — but there's no way we're getting into all of that — though it's worth remembering that if the patient is in atrial fibrillation, the JVP should be irregular with no a-wave.

Then:

1 If you see it, great. Put your finger on it to make sure you can 'stop' it (which you can't do with a carotid pulse, which furthermore will be palpable), then measure from a point in the middle of the pulse wave (classically one-third of the way up!) vertically[29] down to the afore-mentioned *sternal angle* (only then I called it the angle of Louis. Maybe that means it's not afore-mentioned. Anyway, it's the same angle. No point in being obtuse).

   It's allowed to be up to 2 … 3 … 4 … 5 (I pick 3 … maybe 4 …) cm above before it's considered to be abnormal.

2 If you don't see it, also great. Welcome to the real world. One never does see it. Not really. But while we established types can just pretend it's where we want it to be, based on the rest of the examination (and the echocardiogram findings), you are now obliged to go chasing it. A JVP you can't see can either be normal or abnormal.

   • *Invisible–normal.* This can be for two reasons. It is actually visible, but you are not expert enough to see it. Not much you can do about that, except perhaps to gently put your finger over the area, producing a swollen column of blood which, after you release your finger, suddenly lets your more focused brain see that it is indeed pulsing (like continuing awareness of the background drums in music after the drummer/percussionist's solo). The other reason for the invisible JVP being normal is that … that *is* normal. In the healthy person it doesn't poke itself up above the clavicle when at 45°. So … we test for the 'hepatojugular *reflux*' or 'hepatojugular *reflex*'. The names remain interchangeable among the non-shibbolethed, but

---

[28] At this point I should really quote the textbooks which justify the ranges in this statement. However, that would risk bringing to this work a veneer of respectability which might mislead the reader.

[29] That is, not along the patient's body, but kind of drawing an imaginary line so you can estimate the vertical distance above the sternal angle.

technically it's not a reflex, unless we're suggesting that garden hoses and bagpipes have reflexes. You press gently (OK — we're going to save lots of rainforests in the long run if we decide that all pressing is gentle unless specified otherwise) on the upper abdomen. Classically on the liver, but it doesn't have to be. You're not squeezing blood out of the liver (bagpipes don't have one), but increasing the intra-abdominal pressure in general. Certainly any tenderness of the liver would suggest you avoid it. This gentle pressure will often result in a JVP hitherto sitting below the clavicle to budge up so that you can see it. Traditionally, this is not a sign of pathology.[30] Indeed, it is a reason for rejoicing. You have just proved that the JVP is not increased and do not need to move on to the manoeuvres described below.

(This traditional view is now being vigorously challenged by some of those pesky cardiologists. They say that the IVC in the normal patient is a fairly flaccid tube which pressing the abdomen compresses, *reducing* the blood return to the heart. Thus pressing the abdomen in normals will *lower* the JVP. Only if the IVC is relatively distended with a failing heart will compressing the abdomen create a pressure wave and raise the JVP. Ergo, hepatojugular reflux is *per se* a sign of pathology. This flies in the face of tradition, but despite this, fails to convince me. Fortunately, the cardiologist who told me this assures me that it is only known to him and a handful of people in the entire continent.)

• *Invisible–abnormal* Again this could be incompetence on your part — a pulse welling up under the ear like a croaking frog which you have not spotted. However, it could also be due to a venous pulse so high that it is above the angle of the jaw with the patient at 45°. So get them to sit up straight, and see if it becomes visible. If still not so, it is unlikely to be raised so much that you still can't see it but not impossible (though you would expect to have found pointers elsewhere to a problem of this magnitude). Depending on how things are going vis-à-vis the examiner's humour at this stage,[31] you may wish to try this manoeuvre. You ask the patient to raise their arm and you look for a 'J'VP in the veins around the cubital fossa and forearm. If found (...?...) you can measure perpendicularly down to the angle of Louis as before, and quote this distance to the nearest millimetre to the nearest dumbfounded examiner before ordering some champagne and chocolates.

---

[30] Except ... it sets me wondering. There will normally be mechanisms in place to dilute the effect of the Hep-Jug manoeuvre, and the appearance of the JVP above the clavicle might suggest they are absent or deficient in some way. So its appearance may signify the *absence* of a physiological 'reflex' ... Try saying 'hepatojugular reflex absent!!' next time you watch it pop up in the examiner's face — see what happens.

[31] Not always easy to judge. If they seem jovial, things are almost certainly going well (unless they are real bad mothers). But slightly furrowed brows, inexplicable interest in the weather outside or twiddling with equipment can all be associated with happy or unhappy examiners. Repeated glances at their watch (unless accompanied by a lazy practice golf swing) or constant staring directly in your face are perhaps more worrisome signs. Getting together the next candidate's documentation means you can relax — you're finished, one way or the other.

Pr(a)ecordium[32]

Observation

Our first encounter with one of the basic tenets of clinical examination. Observation before examination. Or, *'look then touch'*. Again one of those irrefutable tenets that doctors themselves rarely follow – well, not literally. The idea behind it is sound. Much information – including negative information – can be gained by simply observing the patient. This includes alerting the observer to potential difficulties with subsequent examination, such as areas which might be tender, or features which might suggest that the patient will have problems moving around or holding certain positions. More positive information might come from scars, dyspnoea at rest, use of accessory muscles, etc. All important stuff. All good reasons to take a good look at the patient, or a particular portion of the patient, before 'moving in'.

It's just that ... well ... it ... kind of looks funny. And the precordium is a fair example. Imagine you're a 30-something female patient. You've helped some 20-year-old guy with a nose-ring to take off all of your upper-body clothing. You sit back (... eventually, after the chump has spent ten minutes insisting for some bizarre reason that you lie at his idea of an angle of 45° – usually around 30°) and now he walks down to the foot of the bed and just stands there, staring at your breasts. Eventually he mutters something along the lines of 'looks OK to me' before fumbling in his pocket for, presumably, a stethoscope.

Doctors usually do the 'observation' bit while the patient and the doctor are preparing for the examination bit. You're settling them back into position, and you're chatting to them, and you're getting ready your stethoscope or whatever and you're taking in information all the time.

Unfortunately, the student/junior doctor examinee is obliged to *show that he is observing*. So this, as well as being an instance when the advice that *the patient is a human* is particularly apposite, is an ideal time to talk through what you are seeing. Even the negatives. Because it lets the patient know what the hell is going on. So mention the absence of dyspnoea[33] ('comfortable at rest') and the absence of scars. Symmetry or asymmetry may, or may not, be an appropriate thing to mention. Any scars that are noted should be described sensitively And are likely to elicit an inquiry from the examiner as to the most likely operation. Know these. Know also that the (mitral) 'valvotomy' scar which loops under the left breast may not be immediately apparent in females, so its existence should be checked for again during further examination. It might even be worthwhile – not so much for your own purposes but for those of the patient – not to notice a scar on first

---

[32] *Praecordium* and *precordium* are essentially interchangeable. In the original Latin, 'prae' means 'in front of' (the heart). English words have used this spelling over the years, but the more modern 'pre' is nowadays used in most formations outside medicine. Thus only those schools happy to be considered archaic would continue to have praefects (or indeed praepostors). One sensible way of striking the balance in walking the tightrope between satisfying correctness and antiquated pedantry in deciding which praefix (see?) to use in such circumstances might involve consulting a quality dictionary such as Chambers and seeing which spelling gives the full spiel and which gets the previously derided 'see elsewhere' treatment. Result in this case 'Prae- – *see* Pre-'. An alternative method, and my own favourite, is to look up an American dictionary and follow the opposite course to any it might suggest.

[33] Technically, a symptom, so we can't see it as a sign. But ...

observation (unless to fail to do so would appear ridiculous). I'm sure that the patient would like to think the scar is not that obvious – certainly not the first thing anyone might notice if looking at their torso. Similarly, I am never embarrassed if I fail to spot that a patient is wearing a wig. Indeed, I usually let them mention it first. Look also for visible pulsations at the apex or more bizarre positions ('dyskinetic segments' we're back at the heart, not the wig).

Examination

Moving from observation to examination requires further acknowledged consent *from the patient*. Sometimes a candidate's obtaining reassurance from the examiner that he or she is allowed to go on to the next stage only highlights their failure to obtain such consent from the patient. Requests for such consent need not be made in any grandiose fashion (indeed such formality often suggests to me that this is also for the examiners' benefit, and while a lot of examination technique is exactly that, consideration for patients should be genuine), but maybe a simple word or two, a gesture even, depending on the candidate's style and their rapport with the patient.

Regardless of the apparent intensity of such rapport, Rule Number 1 for examining the precordium is ... don't touch the nipples. Either of them. This is surprisingly true whether you be examining guys or gals. I am not suggesting this is to an equal extent, but it is an odd sensation for us guys, too.

If, however, you do inadvertently brush the female nipple (and if there was any chance at all that it was advertent you are in the wrong profession – though hopefully not for long), do not panic. Even if this is under exam conditions. Chances are the incident has not been noticed (by the examiner, that is; unless under the influence of 16 different local and general anaesthetics the patient will be acutely aware and her mind will be racing through thoughts of ... what was that? ... was that deliberate? ... is that going to happen again? ... what's my lawyer's number? ...) and it would be an error to draw attention to it. But of course you do have to acknowledge the occurrence to the patient and apologise. This apology, however, is in one respect like that following breaking wind at a cocktail party when only one person has noticed. You are required to apologise to them, but hopefully without anyone else realising that you are apologising – or that you have anything to apologise for. Fortunately, we are always apologising to patients when moving them about, pushing tender bits, catching them with nails (... *fingernails* ... for the umpteenth time this is not a textbook for orthopaedic surgeons), so a simple 'Oh, sorry about that' said sincerely and not too off-handedly whilst going through manoeuvres will usually fail to disturb the slumber of all but the most alert examiner.

You can then carry on defining that indefinable entity – the apex beat. 'The downmost and outermost[34] point where one can feel the prominent/significant/raising two fingers (?!) pulsation of the heart.' Basically it's just the bit where you

---

[34] So what if there's a down-most bit and a separate lateral-most bit? Like going to see the famously most south-westerly point of Europe near Sagres in the Algarve. You walk out to the furthermost tip of Cape Sao Vicente in the pouring wind and (honest) freezing rain and ... there's this other headland which looks about ten feet away sticking out clearly further west and just as clearly still pretty much in Europe, only not so far south ... so ... (sorry, I've forgotten the relevance of any of this ...)

feel the heart beating. Then you have to count down from our ubiquitous[35] angle of Louis (which is at the level of the second rib, not the intercostal space. It is easy to recognise the candidate whose face is transfixed with shock when they for the first time actually do something which they have read about but had previously always changed in their brain so that it seemed to make some sense ...) feeling down the indentations between ribs at the edge of the sternum then outwards to describe it as 'in the fifth intercostal space 1 centimetre lateral to the mid-clavicular line' in *exactly* the same way that you will *never, ever, in your entire life, ever, see an adult doctor do in earnest!!* Just (another) one of those things. If you don't localise the apex beat and define its position you will be hounded mercilessly for the rest of the exam. But your hounder is unlikely to have performed this bizarre ritual in living memory, except to demonstrate its mysteries to other students in order to set them up for the big day.[36] In reality, the hounder will only check for the apex beat to see where to put his stethoscope (or in the case of a cardiologist, echo-jelly).

Meticulous siting of the apex is essentially an affectation. If it is displaced, you'll know. Measuring it will make little difference. Trying to describe the 'character' of the beat seems to me even more ridiculous. 'Heaving' or 'thrusting' – which one's the more turquoise?

One thing worth remembering is the striking statistic, culled from a trustworthy cardiology source,[37] that 50% of the time the apex beat is impalpable. So absolutely no panic is due if you cannot feel it. In fact, rejoice as you do not need to do all that faffing about with the angle of Louis and can simply state that the apex beat is impalpable (probably more precise and acceptable than 'absent'). Be aware, however, that while dextracardia is a very rare phenomenon (1: really quite a lot), like many such features its incidence in exams is demonstrably higher than that.

Right ventricular heave
Flat palm of right hand on left sternal edge with patient breathing out (Why? As we shall see later, breathing *in* should accentuate this phenomenon). Usually you can't feel the heart pumping. If you can, the right ventricle may be hypertrophied or dilated as in mitral stenosis or other causes of pulmonary hypertension. A senior colleague of mine in the past used to insist that this was a *left* ventricular heave. Presumably from learning about it as a left parasternal heave as a youth and the signals getting mixed up some place along the line. No one could dissuade him from this misapprehension, and an entire generation of students were brought up to know that a left parasternal heave signified 'right ventricular hypertrophy ... unless you get Dr XX in the exam, whereupon ...'

Thrills
Flat palm/fingers over valve areas. You may feel the blood flow over a roughened valve (e.g. stenotic) or in a direction it shouldn't (e.g. mitral incompetence). Thrills

---

[35] Bizarre to term something famous for its steadfast-landmark quality as 'ubiquitous', but you know what I mean.

[36] Like a driving instructor telling you to turn right by 'Going *past* the car which is coming in the other direction *also* planning to turn right and **then** turning round the back of him.' Beautiful in concept, but try that when you're driving on the real road and you'll get a mouthful of number-plate.

[37] *Oxymoron* will be dealt with in the glossary.

often feel like a cat's neck when it's purring, so if you've never felt a thrill, make sure you have felt a cat's neck when it's purring. Feeling in the sternal notch often lets you detect an aortic thrill you can't feel over the aortic area itself. If talking your way through the examination, it is worth avoiding the standard statement that you are 'feeling for thrills', as this can be enough to convince an already dubious patient that the exam is a gratuitous assault on their person.

Auscultation

This is a huge subject. The temptation for me to approach it systematically, while against all my instincts, is also huge. Again, I believe a short list of Dos and Don'ts is more appropriate.

Do follow the systematic approach of mitral area, aortic, tricuspid and pulmonary.

Do think about the heart sounds themselves before considering extraneous noises (and extra heart sounds before murmurs).

Don't say 'heart sounds present' unless you can think of a very good reason for them being absent in a non-dead patient. *Do* say something about them (e.g. 'heart sounds normal' or 'soft' or 'first heart sound loud').

Do listen with the patient holding their breath out (this enhances left-sided murmurs) and holding their breath in. *Do not* say that there is no mitral murmur without having put the patient on their left side (... gently ...) breathing out.

Do know why left-sided murmurs are louder breathing out in the first place (it's *not* because the heart is brought closer to the chest wall – well, not sophisti-catedly). Start your clear explanation dealing with breathing *in* first. The decrease in intra-thoracic pressure draws more blood into the right side of the heart, making right-sided murmurs louder. Meantime there is a degree of pooling in the lungs. Then, when you start to breathe out, this pooled blood goes to the left side of the heart, making left-sided murmurs louder during expiration. Basically, the right side of the heart deals with more blood during inspiration, and the left during expiration. This can sometimes help to distinguish a pulmonary murmur from an aortic, or a tricuspid from a mitral.

Do know that the same glib theory explains the accentuation of 'normal' splitting of the second sound during inspiration. Normally the aortic valve closes minimally before the pulmonary, producing between them the 'second heart sound'. Inspiration means more work for the right side and slightly later pulmonary shutting – accentuated in problems that delay this, such as severe pulmonary stenosis or right bundle branch block. 'Reverse splitting' happens in the opposite order, is emphasised in expiration, and occurs if left ventricle outflow is retarded – such as severe aortic stenosis or left bundle branch block. It is rare.

Do remember what I call *McKechnie's Two Rules of Cardiology*.[38]

1   If there is a systolic murmur at the base (aortic area) and at the apex (mitral area), then it is aortic – or there are two murmurs.
2   If you can hear a murmur, then it is systolic (saves all that faffing about with feeling a carotid).

---

[38] For no particular reason, these rules have always reminded me of John Avery's two cardinal rules of wine drinking. 1. Life's too short to drink bad wine. 2. A really *good* bottle of wine is not for a big party, or even a dinner party. No. A *really* good bottle of wine is for two people – or, in an *ideal* world, one.

Do remember that *McKechnie's Rules of Cardiology* — while possessing more than a grain of truth — should be taken with a pinch of salt.[39]

Do think about your findings — both while finding them and while presenting them. Do not present things which make no sense at all — but *do not* change your findings to suit a particular diagnosis that you have decided is correct. It may not be. Certainly for undergraduate exams, many faults in technique or deficiencies in knowledge will be 'let go', but a clearly invented set of findings and diagnosis will give the examiner no option but to mark you down — no matter how pretty you are.[40] And, unusually, to feel no regret or guilt, since clearly your integrity is in question. If you realise that your findings make no sense or are incompatible with Einstein's and others' theories of the universe, *say that* (miss out the bit about Einstein) — and try to work out what might really be happening. A candidate who says that they have found an aortic systolic murmur which they think is aortic stenosis, then points out unprompted that this isn't in keeping with their earlier finding of a collapsing pulse, leading them to wonder if there might be an aortic incompetence murmur which they didn't hear and could they perhaps …? … will fare better than one who plumps for a single finding as being correct and moulds the other findings to suit it.

Do have a quick listen at the lung bases for crackles. *Do* use this opportunity to check for sacral oedema. As with ankles, don't really press for 30 seconds. The guy who said that this demonstrates pathological oedema has never worn socks.

Do bring your own kit. You're familiar with it. You know how to use it. You know that it works. You wouldn't go play the final at Wimbledon with a racquet found lying at the edge of the court — and this is more important. Mess up Wimbledon and they'll still let you play other games of tennis. And wear something that keeps the kit under control. Big dilemma for the ladies.[41] Do you wear a 'proper' (i.e. man-type, with trousers and stuff) suit with pockets you can keep your kit in? Or will that look a bit too power-bimbo? Should you carry a 'handbag', risking the wrath of a Lady Bracknell amongst the examiners? The simple answer to this is … I have no idea. It probably makes no real difference except to your own feelings of confidence about your appearance. A female colleague tells of sitting the 'short cases' in the old Membership exam, taking the different instruments from her bag as she went round — not realising that she was blithely discarding them after use. The 'organising' SHO willingly trotted round after her, presenting her at the end with a stethoscope, a pocket ophthalmoscope, a tomahawk hammer, two hair-pins (one bleeding), one lipstick and a (still-wrapped) condom.

Do use the bell and the diaphragm (… no …). We old guys like to think that the bell is better for low-pitched murmurs, and the diaphragm for higher frequencies. The theory is challenged by the design of the modern tubes, which are essentially all diaphragm, but even these tend to have some little lever you can switch to lift something off something else that apparently makes it work like a bell …

So, at some point, click the lever.

---

[39] McKechnie himself went on to be a radiologist.

[40] OK. Not necessarily true …

[41] It is now generally accepted that 'ladies' is a derogatory term — which I therefore use unadvisedly.

Do buy yourself a decent stethoscope. Think about it. It's your *life* ... and not just yours.

Like the original 'Commandments', the above can be summarised by one piece of advice.

Do be considerate and sensible.

Real life

It is an unavoidable trap that 'textbooks' drift into 'passing exam mode' and much advice concerning looking after real people is omitted — as the situation can't crop up in exams. So:

Left ventricular failure

The three cardinal signs classically are *pulsus alternans, extra heart sound* (gallop rhythm) and *basal crepitations.*

(It is a favourite question of mine to ask for the three cardinal signs and listen as most candidates rhyme off a list of symptoms. *Symptoms* are things that patients feel and complain of. *Signs* are the things that we find during examination. Some features can be both.)

The first sign is in fact rare, since established heart failure soon throws away the *big* pulse ... *little* pulse ... *big* pulse ... effect,[42] but substitute tachycardia and you have a simple triad of signs which makes perfect sense and which everybody ignores. People go around diagnosing LVF on anybody with a few basal crepitations (or 'crackles', as the respiratory guys would have us call them), but unless you are on a beta-blocker or have some odd conduction problem that'll show up on ECG, you can't really have LVF without a tachycardia.

The extra heart sounds themselves become audible with experience. Supposedly a third sound makes the heart's cadence sound like 'Kentu**ky**', whilst a fourth makes it resemble '**Ten**nessee'. To maintain this theme, while my own preferred description of the almost inaudible blowing murmur of aortic incompetence[43] is 'an absence of silence' in diastole, I can see how a case might be made for a *sotto voce* romantic whisper of 'Vir-gin-**iaaaah ...**'

Cardiac management

This is now every bit as easy for the cardiologist as history taking. Billions of dollars spent on research such as the ISIS (International Study of Infarct Survival) studies, the WOSCOPS (**W**est **o**f **S**cotland **Co**ronary **P**revention **S**tudy) and the

---

[42] The glib explanation for pulsus alternans goes like this. Left ventricle with blood in it. Not very good LV will not push out all the blood (*small* pulse), so when filled for the next beat it will contain some extra blood. But this extra will slightly stretch the myocardial fibres, inducing a better contraction (Starling's Law — well, one of them) and so it manages to push out all the blood (*big* pulse). Next beat starts with the smaller volume with consequently poor contraction and small pulse ... and so on. As the problem worsens, Starling's Law is overcome, the heart 'decompensates' and pulsus alternans stops. Thus it is considered a sign of 'early' cardiac failure. Convinced ...?

[43] See *McKechnie's Second Rule of Cardiology.*

EUROPA (**Eu**ropean Trial on **R**eduction **of** Cardiac Events with **P**erindopril in Stable Coronary Artery Disease!!!) led to the pivotal 'All-Cardiac-Remedies-Obviously-Negate-Your-Mortality' meta-analysis (they couldn't think of a nifty title) which happily showed that every single cardiac drug improves either symptoms or mortality *over and above* the effects of all the other drugs. So any patient with IHD or failure is given *all* the treatments by their friendly cardiologist, and you'll find drugs like carvedilol and candesartan being taken by 30-year-old marathon runners who felt a bit breathless as they crossed the tape.

You can never be too careful with these important diseases ...

3

Respiratory medicine

Respiratory physicians are a different breed to cardiologists. They don't drive fast cars, don't buy yachts and don't get invited to all the best cocktail parties.[1]

We have previously touched on the public perception of the heart. It's big, it's important, and they can see why. The heart is basically a pump. Without it, the blood doesn't go around and you die. Simple as that. I suppose there is some disparity here, as the general public doesn't quite heap the same adulation on central heating plumbers as it does on cardiologists (among doctors, the converse is true), but this may be because cardiologists aren't quite so hands-on. Not so much the man cutting the pipes as the engineer who knows how to work those little electronic gadget-boxes designed to ensure that the central heating always comes on at two in the morning, except when it stays on all day every day if you're holidaying in the Algarve. Even that analogy doesn't hang together, since there is no major kudos for the plumber himself, yet oodles for the cardiothoracic surgeon who is, after all, a cardiologist with a spanner.

But, unlike the heart, it's not obvious to Joe Public why the lungs are important, or even how they work. On the one hand we have something that pumps fluid round a big long tube. On the other we have all them gas-exchange mechanisms across interfacing membranes of various semi-permeabilities dependent on pH, altitude and probably which side of the equator you are standing on. Consequently, while cardiologists themselves are simple souls with a direct approach to life ('take this tablet – it'll open up all the blood vessels. And if it doesn't work, I'll blow them all up with a big balloon'), chest physicians are more complex individuals. Complex, but not necessarily exciting. They drive the larger varieties of Volkswagens, 4 × 4s or estate cars, and spend their evenings reading back copies of *Thorax* to the sounds of Classic FM, dreaming of what it might be like at a cocktail party.

It's the diseases, you see. They get them down. But 'twas not always thus. In the old days, there was tuberculosis. A cracking disease. Cut people down in their prime – thin, pale people wasting delicately away (aesthetic asthenia) dropping the occasional pristine gob of crystal-clear haemoptysis on to the piano keyboard. Even the treatments were upmarket – sending people off to chalets in the Swiss Alps where the fresh mountain air would cleanse their lungs, failing which, the snow would at least give an even more dramatic backdrop to those pristine gobs ...

---

[1] There is, of course, no longer such a thing as a cocktail party. But you know what I mean. There is no satisfactory current equivalent phrase – 'drinking party' giving out all the wrong vibes.

Then it all went wrong. Improved social conditions, antibiotics and the BCG jab for schoolchildren[2] conspired so that TB was all but eradicated from the Western world. And, it had to be said, not by respiratory physicians. Despite their feeble claims that TB is making a comeback, the fraternity since that time has been a cast of characters in search of a disease.

And chronic bronchitis is not a glamorous replacement.

Old, wizened subjects … smelling of fags … coughing up large quantities of foul muck … and all the time a nagging, not entirely true subtext that … *it's all their own fault.*

No wonder chest physicians have gone rapidly downhill. Desperately seeking sustenance, many have hitched their wagons to the no more palatable but certainly more publicity-friendly specialty of cancer medicine. The lung oncologist is a new breed, and gives the chest guys a shot at the big bucks for research – since everybody likes to be seen giving money to help 'fight cancer'. Of course, such money is mainly used to send 'cancer-fighters' to huge meetings in faded Mediterranean resorts where they can discuss which of three drugs – each costing £20 000 per month – is most likely to prolong the average survival time of cancer X from 6 months to 6.5 months.[3]

As a rheumatologist,[4] it would be churlish of me to suggest that the money spent researching, producing and supplying the drug that will enable *some* of the sufferers from a particular (tragic) disease to have two extra weeks – mainly spent in a research facility having blood tests done – could probably pay for a walk-in shower with piped quadraphonic hi-fi for every arthritis sufferer in the entire country. So I wont.

Seems worth noting, however, that both charities and governments seem happier spending money trying to prevent the inevitability of death rather than improving the lot of people while they are alive on this planet. Maybe that tells us more about human nature than politics.

Meanwhile, what about our respiratory cancer expert? Personally, I wouldn't give much for his own five-year survival rate, since he is up against arguably the biggest terror which mankind will ever face … the stuff of nightmares … Public Enemy *Numero Uno* …

Oncologists.

The biggest thugs in the business. Mr-Thoughtful-Chest-Person has as much chance of influencing the oncologists' plans as he has of outpacing one of their Boxters in his Volvo Estate.

So what is the ex-TB-repairman to do to get his kicks? Well, a lot of them turn to management, where their complex–organised approach can be quite useful.[5]

---

[2] Initially given at 6 months of age, but later changed to 14 years since the infants were unable to wander around yelling 'watch my BCG!!' to anyone straying within 40 feet of them.

[3] Students of English (who shouldn't be reading this book in the first place) might feel that this sentence is poorly constructed, as it is *the patient with the cancer* whose survival rate they are interested in. However, we don't really want the cancer to survive. More advanced students may see deeper and realise it's some sophisticated metonymous figure-of-speech thing.

[4] The term 'Cinderella specialties' is usually avoided by those of us who are actually in one, though the idea of oncologists as 'Ugly Cysters' does have some appeal.

[5] The same men who can spend years discussing whether the added sounds in the lungs are *râles* (French for 'added sounds in the lungs') or *rhonchi* (sort of Latin for added sounds in the lungs. Might actually be Greek, but given a Latin ending so that it's easier to understand. I think Greek

But others will make teaching their big thing. So if you get a chest physician as an examiner, be aware that he's a more formidable opponent than the cardiologist. If you get an oncologist, kick him on the shins – it's all they understand.

History – acute

A cornucopia of failed approaches

Respiratory medicine is more complicated than cardiac medicine, so it follows that respiratory history taking is more complicated than cardiac. Mainly because there are more than two symptoms. There are three.[6] This complicates things so much that it is impossible to present any sort of simple structured approach.

Watch.

Acute pulmonary diseases: approach 1 – the symptoms

Again, pain and breathlessness are the mainstays. We've already touched on these under cardiac problems so what's new?

Well, *pain* in lung disease is more often the 'pleuritic' type – sharp, increasing with deep inspiration and miserable when you cough. Usually localised to one side.[7] Since the pleura is the site of pretty much every acute lung-induced pain,[8] this doesn't really help you tell pneumonia from pulmonary embolism from pneumothorax. And since musculoskeletal pains (e.g. from a cracked rib) can imitate it, don't use the phrase 'pleuritic pain' with too much diagnostic certainty. Possibly it is best not to use it at all. Again, when taking the history, don't 'lead the witness'. I usually ask if taking a deep breath *helps* the pain at all – the patient's indignant reply to the contrary carrying more conviction than simple agreement with the opposite suggestion. What the patient was doing when the pain started is again important, but so is what they did in the few hours before it. Unaccustomed DIY in women, or carrying shopping-bags in men, can be enough to set off muscular pains which can be difficult to categorise as trivial.

Dyspnoea can safely be called 'breathlessness' within the earshot of respiratory physicians. Pronunciation therefore becomes more a test of sobriety than of ambition. Try to find out if any breathlessness (even writing it is tricky) is really such, or whether it is a difficulty in breathing because of pain. I say 'try', as usually patients can't tell. The third possibility is *hyperventilation*. Patients think that they are breathless but are actually overbreathing. Clues may include their having paraesthesia in the fingers – more helpfully specific if it's round the

---

would pluralise a word by adding an 's' which might confuse a medical person.) find themselves very much at home speaking of '*robust*' '*parameters*' of '*outcome*' and '*process*' measurements.

[6] I have since been informed that the official respiratory line is that there are six: dyspnoea, wheeze, cough, spit, haemoptysis and pain. These guys *count* these things!

[7] Similar pain occurring centrally and anteriorly can be pericarditis – the same rubbing of one inflamed membrane against another inflamed membrane being exacerbated by breathing movements. Pericarditis may be relieved by leaning forward. It perhaps should be mentioned under cardiology, but since cardiologists will deny knowledge of its existence as something they should be looking after, I mention it here.

[8] The pain of bronchial carcinoma – usually a late sign of the disease – is a deep, boring pain gradually coming to the sufferer's attention and then never letting go.

mouth – which may even go on to 'carpal spasm'.[9] This bizarre 'paralysis' locks your fingers stiffly towards your wrist as if you're trying to do a shadow-picture of a swan. It's due to the altered calcium ionisation (important to muscular con-traction – true hypocalcaemia causes a similar sign) in the alkalosis caused by overbreathing. The alkalosis is due to the ridiculous efficiency of 'blowing off CO_2' which we will discuss later. All that acid–base, H^+, CO_2, HCO_3^- stuff makes you alkalotic. That's why diabetic ketoacidosis patients overbreathe like maniacs ('Kussmaul' breathing) in an attempt to combat the acidosis. Standard therapy for hyperventilation is to get the patient to re-breathe expired air – traditionally using a brown paper bag.

Cough
What can I tell you? The 'not-bringing-anything-up' or 'dry' cough might make us think of simple viral *upper respiratory tract infection* (URTI), or perhaps if in bed at night a low-grade asthma or LVF – but we need to make sure we've got the right story. 'Not bringing anything up' might include 'cos I swallow it' or because what they bring up is 'just the usual phlegm'.[10]

Patients are usually quizzical about why we wish to know the colour of said phlegm (particularly if they've just told us they always swallow it). This is amplified when we show specific interest in whether it's white, yellow or green, when the patient knows it's grey. It's always grey. Have you ever seen sputum that wasn't grey? So you've got to look at the sputum yourself to learn anything useful. Among other things, patients will call saliva 'sputum', so 'dirty sputum' could easily mean it was spat up whilst eating black pudding. Therefore, we are required to look at the grey stuff and decide if it's grey-green or grey-yellow or grey-white.

For some reason, asking about haemoptysis never frightens patients as you would expect. 'Any blood in it?' usually meets with a straight yes or no, and you go on to find out if it was mixed in with the spit, whether it was a little drop or big gobs of blood. Paradoxically, the spitting of large quantities of pure blood is *usually* associated with a benign cause – which hard-pressed doctors like myself randomly put down to some small damaged blood vessel somewhere in some old scar tissue with the usual total lack of any evidence. But the small variable bits mixed in are much more sinister.

'Rusty' sputum is a classic for pneumonia … but don't ask me what rusty sputum looks like …

…

What did I tell you?

This isn't working. All over the place. Lacks focus. So next we try looking at the stories of the different diseases and working backwards towards the symptoms.

Acute pulmonary diseases: approach 2 – the diagnoses
- *Pneumonia*: variable-length history of being non-specifically unwell … 'viral' symptoms … then *surprisingly sudden* deterioration, breathlessness (they'll tell you it all started suddenly yesterday afternoon … you have to take them back through the previous few days …), with cough and green or yellow sputum (or … er … rusty …) and pleuritic pain.

---

[9] Almost always referred to as 'carpo-pedal spasm', though no one ever bothers about the feet.
[10] Or 'guitar', as it's known in Glasgow (The Sound of Mucus).

- *Pulmonary embolism*: fairly sudden onset of whole syndrome with shortness of breath and pleuritic pain. Cough with no spit or small quantities not particularly yellow/green ('clear grey'), but occasionally with bits of blood.
- *Pneumothorax*: ridiculously sudden onset of pleuritic pain and breathlessness ... but sometimes, particularly in a small one, there's no breathlessness and it's just the pain ... or occasionally there is no pain and a fast-onset breathlessness is the only clue ... and sometimes it's not that sudden and there's just the dry cough ... sometimes ... or not ...

See? This ain't working either. The answer is clearly the modern mathematical approach. As part of the pretence that medicine is a science and not a craft, the past 30 years have seen moves away from 'experience' as being a physician's main attribute. Information from research is now the ultimate and only way to decide on treatment. *'Evidence-based medicine'* not only has its own title, but its own experts and even its own journal.[11] Accompanying this are the 'systematic' approaches to medical diagnosis. The most ridiculous of these was the 'clinical algorithm' much in vogue in the 1980s and not yet entirely fallen from favour. For these, we pretend that a computeresque pathway, using a flowchart with yes/no responses to questions, can guide us to the correct diagnosis. The assertion that 30 years of experience are no match for a mathematical formula devised by someone at the other end of the country lives on in the current fascination with protocols and guidelines.

Protocols and guidelines

Let's take a brief time-out to analyse that current fascination, which to my mind makes two incorrect assumptions.

Assumption 1 is that every patient and their problems can be categorised, pigeon-holed ... whatever, such that a programmed approach can cope with everything their diseases can throw at you. Like suggesting you could make a protocol for playing cricket[12] – to deal with every ball. *'Take one step forward and hit it ... if it bounces early, step back again and hit it ... if the ball moves to the right then shuffle your left foot back and ... if it swings in the air, then ... or maybe spins up off the ground in the opposite ... er ... you ... and it's going much faster than you first thought ... em ... errr ... adjust ... .'*

It doesn't work. All patients are different and you need to deal with their differences. 'Treat every ball on its merits.' Our protocol *could* tell the young batsman to take one step forward and hit smoothly through the line of the stumps. Then 50% of the time he'll hit the ball fine, 30% of the time it'll fly harmlessly past, and only 20% of the time will he be ... out.

And maybe that's OK – for a useless batsman. And thus we come to *Assumption 2*. Protocols assume that the doctor him- or herself is stupid and useless. A protocol is for useless people to do things *all right*. They can never get you to do things *well*. They presume that a bunch of guys round a table some years ago have a better idea how to treat this patient in front of you right this moment than you do. Despite never having seen them or any results. How bizarre! And what an insult!

---

[11] Which does rather provoke the question – what are all the other journals reporting?
[12] We Scots love cricket analogies – it shows off our cosmopolitan nature.

There is one difference between these two ssumptions. The first will never be correct – patients can never be pigeon-holed. But the second can make itself so. Make doctors use protocols and you can make them stupid and useless. Our guys follow a protocol for the treatment of diabetic ketoacidosis. Because it's there, they feel no need to understand what is actually happening in this situation. So they make no effort to find out. After six months of protocol following, you can ask the simplest question (e.g. about what's happening to potassium), and they'll have no idea.

But let's return to our mathematical approach to chest history taking. We try tabulating the relative associations of each diagnosis with each element of the symptoms, from 1 = most to 3 = least.

	Suddenness of pain	Soreness of pain	Shortness of breath	Dryness of cough
1	Pneumothorax	Pneumothorax	Pneumothorax	Pneumothorax
2	PTE	PTE	PTE	PTE
3	Pneumonia	Pneumonia	Pneumonia	Pneumonia

And, surprisingly, we find that they are all going in the one direction. So the simple answer is:

Acute pulmonary diseases: approach 3 – the *Cosmopolitan* questionnaire
'How Sexy is Your Chest Disease?'[13] (Now that's what I call a ... cute pain!)

1 How sudden was your pain?
   a) Very
   b) Quite
   c) Not very
2 How short of breath are you?
   a) Very
   b) Quite
   c) Not very
3 How sore is the pain?
   a) Very
   b) Quite
   c) Not very
4 How dry is your cough?
   a) Very
   b) Quite
   c) Not very

How did you do?
If you scored mainly a's then you have a pneumothorax and should have a tube put into your chest right away. If you were a high b scorer, then you have had a

---

[13] This title is in no way misleading. It is well recognised that any *Cosmo* article headlined with the words 'sexy', 'erotic' or 'lust' will not contain any more references to these concepts in the actual text. (I remain unsure where best to place 'frustratingly' in that sentence.)

pulmonary embolism and should take rat poison. If mainly c's are your bag, then it's a pneumonia and you require an antibiotic. If your answers are a mixture, then you should probably see a doctor, but since protocols are infallible it is likely that there is nothing wrong with you and you should learn to get out more. Perhaps you and your partner could take up salsa lessons ...

History – chronic

Let's stick with the disease-orientated approach.

Chronic obstructive pulmonary disease (COPD)

Another example of the respiratory physicians' penchant for changing the names of things. COA(irways)D was already a change of title for *two* diseases – chronic bronchitis and emphysema. The former was classically a diagnosis from history, where three (or was it two?) consecutive years of two (or was it three?) months (or was it weeks?) of continual productive cough for no good reason meant that you had chronic bronchitis. Emphysema was a 'pathological' diagnosis – the millions of tiny alveoli coalescing into lesser millions of bigger bags making gas transfer less efficient could only be confirmed histologically, though an X-ray will occasionally show stupidly large bags – or at least 'hyperexpanded' lungs spanning more ribs than normal, and spreading flat the diaphragm.

Both were due to smoking. Despite the resultant forms of respiratory failure being at opposite ends of the spectrum – chronic bronchitis causing a CO_2-retention type ('blue-bloater') and emphysema a low CO_2 type ('pink-puffer') – the expert-specialist-heroes inexplicably found them more and more difficult to tell apart until the two diseases were lumped together as COAD. This despite the fact that oxygen treatment is also entirely different in the two scenarios. A 'CO_2-retainer' (blue-bloater) is in danger if given high-percentage oxygen.[14] It works like this. Breathing is driven by two factors sensed by the body – high CO_2 or low O_2. Either situation makes you breathe harder. If your CO_2 becomes persistently high, some people's brains decide to ignore this after a while and will only speed up breathing if the oxygen concentration starts to fall. So if you give high-flow oxygen, artificially keeping up the blood oxygen, they'll hardly bother to breathe ... they won't 'blow off' CO_2, and their blood CO_2 levels will rise. The brain ignores this, taking the occasional breath of the pure oxygen to keep the blood oxygen at some OK level. People seem to think 'that's OK, they'll still breathe if a low oxygen says they have to ...', but the rising CO_2 is itself toxic. Hypercapnia[15] will eventually cause an abrupt respiratory arrest and ... death. So you need to avoid high-flow oxygen in CO_2-retainers – a fact not always appreciated by ambulancemen (and indeed Accident and Emergency staff), who tend to treat all breathing problems as if they were 20-year-old athletes with chest wounds.

---

[14] Have got fed up searching the subscript toggle, so you'll just have to be aware that O_2 is the same as oxygen. See. Don't tell anyone this book taught you nothing.

[15] The occasional ingénue will write this as hypercapnoea making sense only if the patient was being over-managed with the brown paper bag in hyperventilation (*see above*) or was an unlucky astronaut. You'll note it's a mistake unlikely to be made by those who pronounce 'dyspnoea' properly.

(Always check that potential CO_2-retainers have the right sort of mask. People get really sloppy with O_2 therapy. Ask what percentage O_2 the patient is getting and nine times out of ten you'll be told 'two litres' or 'four litres' as if that were a percentage. Trauma masks and Hudson masks will usually give too much oxygen to COPD patients. And don't believe the first nurse/casualty officer/salesman who tells you that *this mask* is OK. They always tell you that. They think air gets magically into any mask, just because it's see-through. You want *lots of holes* in the piping.)

Meanwhile, back at the lunch for deciding nomenclature, further negotiations led to a further change – the 'airways' becoming 'pulmonary'. COAD became COPD. This did mean that a permanently blocked nose could no longer be categorised as COAD, so they may have had a point.

One important thing to remember about COAD (OK, other than the fact that it is now COPD ... I forgot ...) is that you cannot diagnose it on chest X-ray – until you are over the age of 32. It is an established dogma of radiology teaching that COPD causes no changes on the chest X-ray, but a brief review of film reports by consultant radiologists will reveal frequent references to the 'changes of COPD' or 'changes compatible with COPD'.

The 'compatible with' does, of course, allow for the fact that there are indeed no changes one would associate with COPD. The phrase itself perhaps requires analysis. Radiologists insist that we give them as much clinical information as possible on a request form – some departments have even gone to the level of refusing requests which are not satisfactorily completed. The information is to facilitate their reporting, ostensibly to focus their attention in the appropriate direction. Such information is an extremely bad idea. It is self-evident that you get a more unbiased view of an X-ray – or of anything – if you have no preconceived notions. Once you give a radiologist a likely diagnosis, his mind is set in that direction and it will take pretty clamant signs to redivert it. If you suggest '?rheumatoid arthritis' on the form, you might get a report saying 'compatible with rheumatoid arthritis' even if there is no way that it would be the first thing they would think of.[16] The X-ray report therefore gives you less information than it would otherwise. I say let them tell you what they see 'blind', and then you can add this information to your clinical findings. So:

Heresy Tip No. 3   Do not put any clinical details that are likely to influence a radiological report on the request card.

Heresy Tip No. 4   Same goes for histology: *'findings are consistent with the presumed diagnosis of non-specific connective tissue disease ...'* – what is the point?

---

[16] At one stage, local assessment of V/Q scans for pulmonary embolism took this to extremes where pointers from the clinical history were processed into the radiological report. Thus their opinion on 'moderate probability of PTE', etc. included the evidence that the clinician was already considering, such as the nature of the pain, to ask for the test in the first place.

Pulmonary fibrosis

Progressive breathlessness initially on major exertion and gradually occurring on less and less effort. Occupational history becomes hugely important in this scenario. The relevant features are forever changing. Coal miners are becoming scarcer – maple-bark strippers arguably more so – but asbestos exposure remains an important pointer, particularly as in the UK there is financial compensation for those made ill by previous exposure to asbestos. It's important to make the connection for the benefit of the patient and their dependents.

Respiratory failure

This was briefly referred to above. There are two types, cleverly termed Type 1 and Type 2. In both, the oxygen saturation in the blood is decreased. In Type 1, the CO_2 is normal/decreased, and in Type 2 it is increased.

Exam Tip No. 1   If asked to explain the difference, or how it comes about, remember two things:

1   CO_2 crosses the membrane-thingies between blood and air much more easily than O_2.
2   *Do not use COPD as your example for illustration.*

Let me explain. The best example to use for Type 1 respiratory failure is pulmonary embolism/infarct. A small thrombus clogs up a pulmonary artery so that its perfusion area receives no blood. The V/Q scan is the classic test for this, and shows areas of the lung where there is no perfusion (i.e. no blood getting there) but the lung is ventilated normally. Since CO_2 crosses the barriers more easily, the patient manages to blow this off well enough in the areas that are both perfused and ventilated. But in these now limited areas not enough oxygen is getting transferred, so they try to breathe a bit harder. This brings the O_2 up towards normal, meanwhile *blowing off even more CO_2 than strictly necessary*, so the CO_2 levels become *low*.

The best example to use for Type 2 respiratory failure is the (rare) opiate intoxication. The patient simply breathes less than he ought to. The lung is ventilated less than it ought to be, and the patient simply fails to either blow off enough CO_2 or maintain his O_2.

But *don't* try to explain either type using COPD. It seems to start off OK. 'Bronchitis – clogged up/obstructed air tubes … not enough air gets in … lungs don't perform either function …' … but then one examiner points out that asthma is also obstructive, so why does it give you Type 1? … and you have to say 'oooh, maybe not all the tubes are constricted and enough air gets in to allow you to blow off CO_2 – which is, of course, easier (you add confidently) … ' … at which point your other interrogator throws emphysema at you … why is it different from chronic bronchitis? … (particularly since the respiratory chappies have now decided they're the same disease) … ? … and you say … could I … possibly? … phone a friend? …

Use the pulmonary embolism and opiate toxicity.

Bronchial carcinoma

Sufferers may have pain – not usually pleuritic ... gradually worsening, and may have haemoptysis ... small bits mixed into sputum, and may have increasing dyspnoea ... The bottom line is that for *any* pulmonary symptoms plus *weight loss* in a patient who smokes you must at least suspect bronchial carcinoma. This scenario also does for tuberculosis. Particularly if the smoking isn't there, or if there's a hint of night-time fevers, TB needs to be excluded.

(Cynical)[17] Tip No. 5   It's more important to chase an unlikely diagnosis which you can do something about than to chase a more likely one which is entirely untreatable.
Or:
Just because the scan findings are ten times more likely to be metastatic carcinoma than metastatic TB doesn't mean you can't make a case for anti-TB therapy.

Smoking

No matter how we try to schematise the history taking in respiratory disease, we can't ignore smoking. It makes almost all pulmonary disease more likely (though you could argue that this makes it less helpful as a diagnostic pointer). Indeed it makes most diseases in most places more likely. There have been some suggestions for diseases that are *less* likely to occur in smokers. The observed decreased incidence of ulcerative colitis, however, was later paralleled by an increase in Crohn's disease, leading to suggestions that smoking may simply influence the form of your inflammatory bowel disease. It may not be as simple as that. An oddly similar scenario is a possible association of smoking with a decreased incidence of endometrial carcinoma, but increased cervical carcinoma. Another suggestion, that DVTs were less likely in smokers, disappeared from view without explanation, and to date the only condition with which we can confidently predict a negative association appears to be longevity.

This predictive value for so many diseases has led to calls for some sort of sanctions against smokers – such as charging them for treatment. I may be cynical, but I can spot this as nonsense. We don't refuse to treat a footballer's broken leg because he continues to play football. Even an amateur tightrope walker would merit treatment as per usual.[18] Smokers do, however, see their own habit as carrying some stigma (they are the ones who will usually voice aloud that 'it's my own fault'). This can make obtaining an accurate appraisal of cigarette intake tricky, as they do not wish to appear undeserving of our attentions. There is a 'conventional wisdom' that you should take the figure they offer you and double it. Patients are becoming aware of this. Recently one told me 'I know you doctors

---

[17] Not entirely convinced this is cynical.
[18] Though you wouldn't expect him to deny the likely cause of his injuries ... 'Why has this happened to *me*?' ... or meet suggestions he might try walking fewer tightropes with ... 'easier said than done'.

will just take the number I say and double it, but I *really do* smoke 10 a day'. My subliminal response was to realise that since he knew I'd double the figure, he was suggesting 10 knowing that this meant 20. Therefore my subthalamus doubled *this* figure and I decided that he smoked 40 per day.

> **Cynical Tip No. 6** When asking a patient how many cigarettes they smoke, also ask if they have heard that doctors automatically double this figure. If they have, quadruple it.

Ex-smokers may also be similarly vague about when they gave up.

> 'Do you smoke cigarettes, Mr Smith?'
> 'Naw — but ah used to smoke at one time.'
> '. . . and when was it you stopped?'
> '. . . Tuesday[19].'

Cigarette-smoking is another avenue for those who like to quantify things. More and more I'm seeing smoking history described in the clerk-in as '30 pack years' or somesuch. While this is appropriate for research, it lacks the feel of a brief description of someone's smoking career. Its predictive ability may also be less than suggested. A pack a day for the last 30 years probably predicts current problems differently from a 30-pack-a-day smoke-fest in 1967.

Family history

My respiratory colleagues insist that I mention this. A family history of 'atopy' (weird word — always seems like there's a bit missing) is associated with asthma. A family history of TB is associated with … TB. But family history is a double-edged sword — it can take you down the wrong path,[20] particularly if the patient has already taken the first steps.

Examination

General

It is usual to assess whether you feel that the patient is 'comfortable' with their breathing at rest. Again, some attempts at quantifying this have been made — mainly with the potential observation that the patient is using their 'accessory muscles' to assist breathing. Personally I have no idea which muscles these are, but it certainly is the case that struggling patients seem to use neck movements in an attempt to help their respiration. Normal breathing is done at the diaphragmatic level. It moves down, the chest is expanded, the pressure inside is reduced and air is 'sucked' in. We only start to use thoracic (muscle) breathing when under some

---

[19] The day of admission. True story.
[20] OK. If we did want to avoid the mixed metaphor, just how were we going to develop the sword image?

stress, or looking for 'that bit extra'. I can only assume that using neck muscles is the next step in thoracic breathing[21] and denotes a further stage in the struggling.

Hands

Cyanosis

Cyanosis is a blueish tinge of the tissues usually noted in the tongue and lips (central[22]) or in the fingers/toes or even hands/feet (peripheral). This blueness can often be overlooked as we get used to patients 'looking like that'. Students who state that there is no cyanosis are often surprised if they are encouraged to compare the patient's lip colour with that of one of their young colleagues (or even my own, to prove that it isn't just an age thing, though oddly this is becoming less convincing ...).

Before we go into the vagaries of 'central' and 'peripheral', let's deal with what the blueness itself signifies. Blood is red because oxygenated haemoglobin is red. Deoxygenated haemoglobin is more of a blue colour (veins vs. arteries!), so the blueish tinge is due to increased deoxygenated haemoglobin in the blood. I like to use the scientific term for deoxygenated – 'reduced' (as in Red/Ox equations – remember schoolday mnemonics like 'Loss of Electrons = Oxidation'?) – if only so that I can say cyanosis is due to 'increased reduced haemoglobin'.

Now comes the brilliant trick question.

What percentage of your haemoglobin has to be reduced to give you cyanosis?

You can even tell people it's a trick question (only fair). Only after crazy guesses from 5% to 95%[23] will some bright spark realise that it's not a percentage, but an absolute concentration. The first bright spark who noticed this guessed the required concentration of reduced haemoglobin to be about 5 g/dL (50 g/L), and this figure has rather stuck – though the truth is closer to 3.5 g/dL. But the realisation that *it is not a percentage* is the key. Thus patients with anaemia (despite this condition being a favourite response to 'causes of cyanosis? ... ') do *not* get cyanosed (think about it – if your haemoglobin is 6 g/dL, what are your chances of survival if 3.5–5 g/dL is deoxygenated?), while people with polycythaemia – with haemoglobin levels up at 20 g/dL – will very likely appear cyanosed even if they are keeping rather well.

---

[21] As you probably know, operatic singers are taught to use diaphragmatic breathing at all times – despite the natural tendency to adopt thoracic breathing under the 'stress' of trying to sing – as this 'improves control'. To be honest, I have never been convinced as to whether this is genuine or simply a centuries-old ruse conjured up by singing teachers so that they have something to teach. It probably seems easier to justify ten years of weekly sessions teaching 'breath control' than 'how high the correct notes are' to someone who can already *hear*. (Author's note: now I come to reconsider this statement, *nothing* seems less justifiable than the concept of teaching someone to breathe.) What I haven't previously considered is whether years of such training will abolish the 'accessory muscle sign' in opera singers – who will doggedly stick to diaphragmatic technique while breathing their last. Would Mimi have survived her tuberculosis long enough for antibiotics to be invented if she'd just tried gasping like the rest of us?

[22] There has been recent speculation that cyanosis of the lips is peripheral, and that only the tongue is truly central. This seems to take rather a simplistic view of the periphery in the absence of an 'end-artery' effect at the lips, even though they are more exposed to the outside cold. Certainly my own view would be that blue lips in a warm room suggest *central* cyanosis.

[23] Budding football managers may suggest 110%.

'Peripheral' and 'central' cyanosis can cause further confusion. If a patient has blue fingers, is that peripheral or central cyanosis? The answer is that you don't know. Peripheral cyanosis occurs when there is some peripheral problem in the circulation and this might well cause blue fingers (if that is the area involved), but if you have problems with your heart and lungs – the areas that cause central cyanosis and blue tongue/lips – there is no process which magically prevents your fingers from also being blue. So blue fingers could be due to either central or peripheral cyanosis. I like to call the sign 'cyanosis in the periphery' to distinguish it from the 'diagnostic' term 'peripheral cyanosis'. On finding blue fingers, we are obliged to inspect the tongue to determine which form of cyanosis is present.

Having said the above, it's worth noting that a cold blue hand is likely to be peripheral cyanosis, while a warm blue hand is more likely to be central. Thus if given a blue hand to examine and nothing else,[24] you could at least hazard a guess at the nature of the cyanosis.

Clubbing

We have dealt with the elucidation of clubbing elsewhere. Respiratory causes are legion and severely test this book's aspiration to avoid 'lists'. Let us simply state that clubbing is clearly a chronic phenomenon. Pulmonary embolism, pneumonia and pneumothorax will therefore *not* be associated with clubbing (excluding any untoward incident at *Stringfellows*). Of the chronic respiratory diseases, COPD, asthma and Wegener's granulomatosis are also *not* associated with clubbing. As for all the others … ?

There we have it. A non-exhaustive non-list.

Other features in the hands include the warm hands with large-volume pulse of hypercapnia, occasionally accompanied by a 'flapping tremor'. This is demonstrated by having the patient hold their hands out, palms down, and then bend the wrists up. The tremor is more of a twitch than a flap really – an intermittent brief loss of the ability to keep the wrist extended. Indeed the technical term – 'asterixis' – somehow gives a better onomatopoeia for the jerking movement in the hands.

Perhaps the most obvious finding is usually the telltale signs of cigarette smoking. This was called 'nicotine staining' for many years. Deep down, we all knew that nicotine was colourless[25], but only when the general public learned that tobacco contained 'tar' in significant quantities were we able to move to the more

---

[24] Not so unlikely as it might appear. A story used to tour Glasgow Medical Society of professors baiting neonate professors (yes – they have their own hierarchy) by having a patient put their hand through a doorway and the neonate professor on the other side, unable to see the entire patient or ask questions, was obliged to produce a spot diagnosis. On becoming establishment professors themselves, the victims immediately deny all such rumours as ridiculous, while secretly lamenting the passing of these humiliating rituals in our (slightly) more enlightened times.

[25] A similar scenario to the frequent description of a patient 'smelling of alcohol'. Reputedly, lawyers have in the past forced medical practitioners making such a statement to read from a dictionary where alcohol is described as a 'volatile, odourless substance …'. It is of course mainly the odour of breakdown products that we associate with someone having been drinking. The lawyer's ruse works if the doctor, not having encountered this before, allows him- or herself to be rattled. However, much like during clinical exams when we are thrown by a simple concept we haven't bothered to consider before, common sense will usually prevail. I would expect a polite explanation that he 'smelled the way I associate with people who have been drinking alcohol' would be sufficient. The jury will understand. No one as yet insists that we write 'smelling of aldehydes' in the case sheet.

accurate description (though nicotine may 'turn brown on exposure to air') of 'tar staining'. Despite its widespread acceptance, I've yet to see attempts to market Tar Chewing Gum (dosing might be tricky – how many bit-u-meant to eat?), but I'm sure an advertising campaign promising 'authentic teeth-staining without all that mucking about with matches' could soon catch on.

A nice opportunity to impress the patient may occur if they have given up smoking in the recent past. Tar staining on the nails will stop and new nail growth at the cuticle will be clean. The position of the resultant line on the nail will give you some idea how long ago the patient gave up smoking – since it takes 6–9 months for the full regrowth of a fingernail. The effect of glancing at a patient's hands and saying 'so you gave up smoking three months ago' can be quite gratifying.

Chest

A few things we have to do first.

Position of trachea
It is above the supra-sternal notch. The same smart-alec place we felt for an aortic thrill. One finger, two, whatever you like – just don't push too hard. It's a bit sensitive around there. If you feel the trachea and you think it might not be central, then it's central. Significantly displaced tracheae (?) either seem to be in a stupid position, making you unsure whether it is indeed the trachea – or you have trouble finding them at all.

Lymph nodes
You can either do them at the start or at the end of chest examination – the secret, as with many other such things, is always to do them at the same stage. That way you never forget. One thing which always catches the examiner's jaundiced eye – or makes a hitherto glinting eye jaundiced – is the candidate who appears uncertain what to do next. This immediately suggests that they don't examine patients all that often, as otherwise they would automatically move on to whatever it is they always move on to at this point. So the more times you examine patients properly, not only the better you will become, but also the better you will *look*.

Examine for lymph nodes from behind the patient who is sitting up. Start high up behind the ears and work your way down to the supra-clavicular fossae – and really feel for them. Don't go through the motions. Always assume that there are lymph nodes there, and you have to find out where. It's a bit like being a slip-fielder in cricket. Ninety-nine times in a hundred the ball goes nowhere near you, but you must set yourself up for every bowl thinking 'this is the one' and the ball is about to come crashing your way. You must have that mental set with lymph nodes.[26] Use this opportunity to also feel for a goitre – otherwise you'll have to

---

[26] Apologies are required to the distaff side at this point. Not for another cricketing analogy (taken directly from the *MCC Coaching Manual c.*1980), but pre-emptive apologies for my now suggesting that the ladies will not understand it ... and proffering this cheeky alternative: it's like always being aware that this might be *the very stitch* where the whole pattern changes ... and for my Scots brethren who may also be struggling, a 'golfing' analogy ... think of it as being continuously aware that the next round might be yours. ......

pretend there's such a thing as an 'endocrine examination'. The thyroid is exactly where you'd expect it to be, and most patients can manage just the one swallow without actually having anything to drink. All palpable goitres feel asymmetrical to me. Hard cragginess is much more worrying.

Some people dispute whether examination for axillary lymph nodes should be included here. I think it should, as there is no other obvious time, and it would appear foolish to forget it because 'well ... it's not really respiratory, is it? ...'. The technique that I was taught was to get the patient to stretch their arm out, you put your hand up into their axilla, then get them to bring their arm back into a neutral relaxed position. Then you feel around the relaxed armpit. Dead easy. No sweat.

Chest examination: the chest

Ah! Another dilemma. Front or back? The problem here is that we spend our lives examining lungs from the back, but under exam conditions you are suddenly aware of the inadequacies of this approach (e.g. right middle lobe signs might be exclusively audible/percussible from the front) and set about doing all sorts of examinations from alien angles ... percussing a huge worryingly dull mass in the centre of the chest (for which only your fourth suggested differential diagnosis ... *maybe it's the heart!* ... comes up trumps) ... tapping around floppy breasts (those nipples again) ... listening in areas we never listen in – including near to the trachea where all breathing sounds suspiciously bronchial. Maybe it would be best if we were all honest and examined the lungs from the back first, before moving on to the front of the chest afterwards. That way, if the posterior approach reveals all the relevant information, the examiner can interrupt your efforts, and his own ennui, after you have finished the back – as long as you make that 'I-was-just-about-to-examine-the-front' gesture before resigning yourself sulkily to missing it out.

(A footnote [but too large for a footnote ...] occurs to me on the re-mention of nipples. In the real world, it's interesting to note just how much regard for personal space we do [correctly] adopt. Despite conceptually examining the heart before the lungs, I now realise that I almost always examine the back of the chest first – particularly in female patients, as this seems a more gentle and gradual move into the more intrusive parts of physical examination. A famous medical teacher[27] once described a good physical examination as 'like a caress'. While this is rather fanciful,[28] and nowadays maybe actionable,[29] perhaps the 'rules of engagement' of a caress do indeed apply, and one continues clinical examination on an 'if-that-was-OK-then-I'll-do-this-if-that's-OK' basis. A cardiology colleague has recently assuaged my conscience by admitting that he also tends to examine female hearts with the bra still attached – something we will thoroughly frown upon in examinations. There may be an odd ethical point here. As we become more aware of patients' sensitivities, do we become less good at examining them

---

[27] Unfortunately, I can't remember who. Attempts on Google with 'medical examination' plus 'like a caress' have not been successful, and may well land me in trouble ...
[28] I genuinely wrote this in my first draft as 'fanciable' – any Freud fans out there?
[29] And this read much better when the previous was 'fanciable'.

for abnormalities? As a consequence, in the case of chest examination, do women get examined less thoroughly than men?)

So, examination of the chest:

Observation again. Looking for big looping scars from removal of lungs or of lobes of lungs (why do they all look the same size?) and any areas of non-expansion or reduced expansion before touching the patient.

Chest expansion

Lots of ways to do this – none of them any good. The trick is to use which-ever method you choose *honestly* and get a real feel for how much each lung is expanding under your hand. There is a temptation using standard methods to move the midline thumbs apart as the patient breathes in, just to show the examiner that your technique works. Resist this. Not only does it make it more difficult for you to feel genuine differences under your fingers, but it often leads to embarrassment when the patient breathes all the way out again, yet your thumbs go nowhere near back to their original position – your realisation of which is followed by surreptitious attempts to make the thumbs gently float together as if the patient is still breathing out ... by which time he is breathing *in* again, but you have your thumbs paradoxically coming together ... which could only suggest to the examiner that the patient has a flail segment from being hit by a passing motor-cycle or ...

Examination Rule No. 3   Never try to deceive the examiner. Tell the truth.

Measuring all-round chest expansion is another quantification bizarreness. You do it by winding a tape-measure round the patient's chest and pulling it tight while they totally breathe out, marking this point, then measuring the difference as they totally breathe in. The bizarreness is not simply that you feel like a tailor (though not so acutely as when doing the 'inside-leg-measurement' manoeuvre for true and false leg shortening[30]), or again the *damned trickiness of the female body* – which is no more designed to facilitate medical examination than are the paper gowns in outpatient clinics – but the measurement itself. Normal chest expansion, we are told, is 5 cm (previously calculated by ourselves as approximately 2 inches). I have seen perhaps two patients in my entire life who have reached this standard. And this is not simply because, like most of the other clinical tests in this book, as a consultant I never bother to do it. In rheumatology we do check chest expansion, as it can be reduced in ankylosing spondylitis (... yes ... good point ... shows you're thinking scientifically ... but my experience does include all the people with *suspected* ankylosing spondylitis plus lots of others I've examined for lots of other reasons).

---

[30] The funniest medical joke ever written in the entire history of the earth concerns inside-leg measurements. It is to be found in Appendix 1, unless it has been removed by the powers that be on the grounds of decency. As already intimated, the removal-of-the-Appendix concept is a recurring second-best-ever medical joke.

A turning-a-blind-eye type of approach has grown up, like the police with cannabis, or referees with pushing and shoving in the box.[31] While everybody quotes 5 cm as the norm, nobody takes any notice unless the chest expansion is below 3 cm.

Percussion

Get used to it. Just do it lots and lots and lots. And don't try any of those half-way-house efforts of using two pleximeter (that's the flat one [usually middle] held on the chest wall) fingers or using two striking (that's the one that ... er ... strikes) fingers. Just keep doing it properly lots of times – and relax!!

At a slightly more refined level, don't leave the striking finger flat on the pleximeter after striking. Pull it back off immediately. It's almost as if you start the draw-back before the finger touches, though overdoing this can look a tad incompetent (see reflex testing).

Another thing to remember is that while a nice clear note is lovely – particularly for demonstration purposes – the *feel* of the resonance is almost as important. Much can often be learned from very light percussion of which no one but the person performing the examination is particularly aware.

And the other other thing to remember is the name Auenbrugger.

Leopold Auenbrugger was the medical student who 'invented' percussion. Reputedly his father was a wine merchant who used the technique to determine the level of wine in his wooden barrels. Auenbrugger Junior, while still a medical student, adapted the idea to determine fluid levels in the lungs of his patients. Hopefully he was severely reprimanded for his smart-alecism.[32]

The normal percussion note in the chest is 'resonant' (get used to the sound). It's reduced in lots of things – consolidation, pleural thickening etc. Pleural effusion does indeed give 'stoney dullness' – immediately recognisable even if you've never actually percussed a stone (but do so sometime – compare the note of percussing a modern particularly plasterboard wall with a proper wall in an old stone building[33]). Increased resonance, to be honest, is difficult to be confident about – but occurs with pneumothorax and emphysema (unilateral – guess pneumothorax; bilateral – guess emphysema).

Vocal fremitus

Only if you've forgotten your stethoscope.

---

[31] The ruination of modern-day football. Everyone pushes and shoves all the time, so it becomes the norm. So when, purely on a whim (or bias, or earlier visit to Ladbrokes), the referee decides to give a penalty, slow-motion replays will always show that there 'was contact' – though the fact that this was the fifteenth contact inside two seconds is ignored along with the unlikelihood of a 13-stone trained professional athlete with muscles on his muscles and nandrolone coming out his ears being sent rolling 15 yards by the touch of a pinkie on his back. Just as well the guys have fancy cars – how would they survive in a Tube station?

[32] The myth that piano players should be good at percussion is actually given some genetic support by the Auenbrugger family, all of Leopold's daughters being accomplished pianists – at the level of having pieces dedicated to them by Haydn.

[33] Arguably my most singular success with percussion was to correctly place the screws for the 'clothes pulley' into the hard wooden joists hidden behind the kitchen ceiling by percussing out their positions. A later effort to repeat the feat reminded me why pleural effusions are 'dull'. They are full of fluid. Just like water-pipes.

Auscultation

Only if you've *not* forgotten your stethoscope (that old 'invasion of personal space' thing again …)

Listen all over, at the same place on each side before moving on. Normal respiration ('vesicular' breath sounds) classically has no space between inspiration and expiration, but the main difference from 'bronchial breathing' is that the expiratory phase is almost silent, whereas in bronchial breath sounds it is, if not harsh, at least obvious. Prolongation of the expiratory phase can be a sign of mild or dormant asthma (or emphysema). Check by asking the patient to breathe out as fast as they can, which brings to the fore any latent wheeze.

Added sounds

Back in the old days 'râles' (from the French word 'râle', which means a râle) was the word for added sounds. These were divided into:

1 wheezing sounds – called 'rhonchi' (singular = rhonchus) when heard via the stethoscope, or simply 'wheeze' when audible at the end of the bed
2 crackling sounds (like rubbing your hair together between your fingers) called 'crepitations'. These were further divided into the 'fine' crepitations of LVF and early interstitial lung disease, and the 'coarse' moister sounds of coarse fibrosis, infection, COPD, etc.

But forget that.

Those nice respiratory chaps have of course been mucking about with these excellent terms, since they are difficult to define, and want us now to call all wheezing sounds 'wheezes' and all crackling sounds … well … 'crackles'. 'Wheezing' therefore no longer distinguishes between a fine wheeze heard on careful auscultation and broken steam-engine noises that would keep you awake at the other end of the ward. This is called 'progress'.

'Stridor' merits a specific mention. It is a wheeze-like noise but caused by obstruction of the upper airways well above the level of the lungs, more prominently inspiratory than wheeze usually is. It may occur with allergic reactions (including anaphylaxis) or other causes of swelling in the throat such as epiglottitis – a rare emergency (one is obliged to mention *ampicillin/amoxycillin* here – just in case it saves one life, one day). A stridor-type noise may also be produced (semi)-voluntarily by the patient under stress or for other reasons.

Cynical Tip No. 7 It may be important to note when apparent wheeze at the bedside is not confirmed by major rhonchi on auscultation, denoting upper respiratory tract noises not particularly suggestive of asthma and not necessarily non-voluntary. A respiratory colleague asks the patient to 'now breathe quietly so that I can listen to the heart sounds' and the wheeze disappears (a wizard wheeze!).

Do listen in the supraclavicular fossae.

Do listen from the front – even if it's only eventually.

Do get the patient to breathe through their mouth. This is not so easy as it sounds. (**Accidental contrariness No. 1**. When asked to breathe through the mouth, almost all patients – especially men, trying to show how rock-hard they are – will immediately start breathing very noisily through the nose (try it and see), and you may have to demonstrate. No particularly deep breathing is required. Indeed a nice, easy, slightly quicker than natural breathing is best.[34])

Do remember that everything is dull/reduced over the scapulae.

Do get the patient to give a cough if you hear a few coarse crepitations – sorry, crackles – at a base to see whether that simple manoeuvre clears them.

Do turn that funny little knob-thing on the stethoscope so that the hole is facing the chest wall.

Vocal resonance (VR)

This supersedes vocal fremitus as it gives the same information arguably more reliably and definitely using the more expensive equipment. (If no stethoscope is available, use the palm of the hand or flat of the ulnar border. This is 'vocal fremitus'.)

Hold the diaphragm of the stethoscope against the chest wall. Ask the patient to say '99' or 'one-one-one' – whichever you come to prefer. Defining normal is again a matter of experience. I like to think that 'normal' sounds as if the '99' is coming from the diaphragm of the stethoscope, 'decreased' sounds as if it's coming from far away, while 'increased' is *in your ears*.

The increased VR in consolidation vs. the more intuitively predictable decrease over an effusion often puzzles people. Explaining that the consolidated lung transmits sound better to the chest wall than open airways starts to make sense, but then the diminished VR over a pleural effusion suddenly becomes problematic. Surely fluid transmits sounds well (even better than air?). Ah yes, but while the boffins tell us that sound travels really well under water (proof for which statement has failed to crop up in my landlubber lifetime), sound travels poorly across the interface between the two media. If you are lying under water, you don't hear much of what's being said above you. Alternatively, sitting sipping a pina colada under your parasol, you don't hear what people are saying at the bottom of the pool (?!). So, since the effusion is outside the lungs and airways themselves, sound doesn't travel well into the effusion, then back out again on to the stethoscope.

Aegophony

This is essentially a variant of increased vocal resonance. Hugely nasal, it does indeed sound like sheep bleating – though for many city-slickers like myself this realisation comes retrospectively and it is many years post medical school before we actually hear a sheep bleat[35] and recognise how apt the description was. We will still be unable to fathom why the tups on a Galloway hillside are saying '99'.

Whispering pectoriloquy is a magic sign. The patient is asked to whisper the ubiquitous '99' while you auscultate. The true fact is that over an area of consolidation you can clearly hear this, but over normal lung you can't. It does rely on

---

[34] Experience of attempting to listen to difficult heart sounds might suggest that the best way to achieve this prominently heard respiration in most patients would be to ask them to 'hold your breath'.

[35] Similar to the 'nutmeg-liver' description from pathology textbooks, supposedly helping generations of students to recognise the hepatic changes of congestive cardiac failure when seen under the microscope. Only in our early thirties, as a 'new man' following our first Nigel Slater recipe, does it make sense when we actually see for the first time the inside of a nutmeg – henceforth known to us as 'Dropsy Spice' (maybe the one axed from the group for not being able to hold her liquor ...).

getting the patient to whisper *properly* (the things we have to teach people!). Most will simply speak quietly when asked to whisper, and this will be conducted as per normal VR. A real whisper (no touching of vocal cords?) is required. Whispering pectoriloquy, along with aegophony and increased VR, are all interrelated signs classically occurring over consolidation, but often are also to be found at the upper border of a pleural effusion. The reason for this is easily explained . . . but not by me.

And that's about it for respiratory examination. We should mention the *peak flow meter'*, a handy tool which can help to define severity – particularly of asthma – as well as helping to monitor the short-term progress of lung disease. The patient is asked to breathe in, wrap their lips round the plastic/cardboard tube and then empty their lungs as fast as they can. No little smarty spit-blows, as this can deceive the machine. The meter records the fastest rate at which the air is expelled at any one point in time (*peak flow*), and part of the fun is to get students to guess the units once they learn that the normal range is about 500–700. So have a guess yourself, then look up the answer in Appendix 2. Then think just how ridiculous your guess was.

Cynical Tip No. 8   Peak flow meters may help to identify if a patient is trying to over-emphasise the level of their dyspnoea (not, of course, that one would suggest that this ever happens). If they genuinely try their best, the result (once they are trained) will be fairly consistent. Results that are 'all over the shop' may suggest a lack of consistent effort.

4

Gastroenterology

If one stops for a moment to consider what they actually do for a living, it's a wonder anyone talks to gastroenterologists at all. At our thematic cocktail party, I have in the past lusted after a more glamorous label to my medical exploits than *rheumatologist*. Joints and stuff.[1] It immediately makes me seem dull and uninteresting – and I like to keep that as some sort of surprise. I've flirted with the idea of telling the thematic cute female that I'm a brain surgeon. It shouldn't be too difficult to bluff one's way through this, in the absence of cute female being a brain surgeon's daughter ('she was only a brain surgeon's daughter, but she knew how to count to ten ...'). And the public do have this rigid pecking order, as we've mentioned before. It's as if they associate the personality of the doctor with the part of the body they work on. So brain surgeons must be extremely clever – 'brainy'. Which brings us back to the opening sentence of this chapter.

Gastroenterology. Hardly the most appealing of specialties for the young up-and-coming ... human. Yet not one that has any problems attracting its adherents. Perhaps they envisage a career dealing with the oesophagus and stomach, and the rest of the gastrointestinal tract gets rather thrust upon them (a sudden image of Laocoön ...). Indeed, if the specialty did divide itself into these two areas (uppers and downers), it might have been interesting to see what sort of characters drifted towards the respective orifices. However, gastroenterology is more far-reaching than this, and practitioners either specialise in *both* of the above (known as lumenologists[2]) or in disorders of the liver (hepatologists). In recent years, the specialty has found itself focusing more and more on the second aspect, a major part of the gastroenterologist's workload now coming from recurrent admissions for alcoholic liver disease.

But let's face it. Their main function is sticking tubes (with 'cameras' or 'telescopes' at the end, depending on what sort of patient you're talking to) up and down people, and overseeing hugely long waiting-lists for these things to prove that the hospital needs another gastroenterologist. In some ways it is the epitome of the 'service' specialty. Physicians seeing patients in general medicine or their own specialty (e.g. rheumatology stalwarts with their anti-inflammatories!) frequently require the help of a gastroenterologist, usually to perform an endoscopy (although it is more polite to disguise this as a request for an opinion). This

[1] At one such 'cocktail party' I was actually asked if I'd ever had to learn any real medicine before going into rheumatology.
[2] Not in any way to be confused with 'luminaries' – though that does spring to mind (... it's a transitive verb, too ...) – the description of an academic gastroenterologist as being like 'a lighthouse in the Sahara'. Brilliant, but totally useless.

'usefulness to others' is a handy attribute when justifying yourself at all sorts of levels. Facilities, funding, extra colleagues, best seat in the coffee room – all are achievable for the practitioner who can offer a service. Bad news for me and my ilk. Respiratory guys supply the occasional bronchoscopy, cardiologists an echo or ETT (though these are likely to be performed by a local schoolkid on work experience while the consultant swans off to examine the Queen's corgis). In my experience, the rheumatologist has less to justify his existence with technician-type requests – joint aspirations being only rarely called for. Granted, there is a move towards enlisting rheumatology help for the all-round-full-assessment-while-pretending-the-problem-might-be-rheumatological sort of diagnostic dilemma, but it's difficult to put these down on paper for the bean counters in NHS management to appreciate.

Clinical pharmacology was worse. It didn't take me long to realise that *nobody* asked you for your opinion[3] – since you had no technical procedure to offer and the last thing a specialist wants to hear is someone else telling him how to use his own favourite drugs.

Thus gastroenterologists have a nice niche. Everyone appreciates them – but they don't have the kudos that might make you envy them. It's a dirty job, but somebody has to do it. Their numbers are therefore made up of generally well-coordinated people who like to be liked, and perhaps even 'like to help others'.[4] Much as a cardiologist likes nothing better than to wade through a busy catheter list, the gastroenterologist revels in immersing him- or herself in all forms of endoscopy sessions – and all that that entails ...

As for cars, it doesn't really matter what they drive, since no one will accept a lift from them in any case. Well, we might as well pretend that someone who works all day in the fish market won't go home smelling of fish. You might think it would make them go for the high-speed freshness of soft-top convertibles, and it may be a local 'Scottish' thing that in my experience they don't – since you only get the chance to keep the top down five days of the year. Is it worth accepting a lift in the pouring rain, knowing you'll be drookit by the time it's finished, just so the driver can pretend they don't work in a fish market?

'I'll give you a run home if you've got an umbrella ... '

History

This time the two symptoms are pain and the nebulous concept of 'bowel habit'. Nice to get rid of dyspnoea finally, but pain again rears its ugly head. Pain. Odd stuff really. We ask the patient where it is, where it goes, what it's like, when they get it (with abdominal pains – whether it's associated with eating or defaecation), what makes it worse ... And all the patient really wants to know is – what'll make it better? Just make it go away and stop asking stupid questions.

What is the point of pain anyway? The usual explanation is that it lets you know there's a problem, and you can protect the area. That works for injuries – the pain

---

[3] Not absolutely true. Advice on the best two-compartmental model to fit the pharmacokinetics of alcohol and its effect on small plastic tubes you might breathe into was occasionally sought.
[4] A characteristic which many of us are trying to eradicate from the medical profession. Despite notable pockets of success – particularly in the afore-mentioned clinical pharmacology and in radiology – we are still well behind schedule. In its own small way, this book may help.

from a sprained ankle effectively tells you not to play football on it (not that you'll listen) – but what's the point of pain in the abdomen? Nothing you can do to protect that. Putting a double tubigrip round your midriff won't cure your ulcer. All that pain really does is let you know something's up and you should go and see your doctor. So the only logical explanation for pain is that God, or Mother Nature, or a simple billion to one chance that was always going to happen without the need for any cosmic intellect, or whoever ... designed the human body to have pain so that sufferers can tell their doctor about it and he or she can make a diagnosis. Pain therefore – despite being a traditional challenge to the existence of an omnipotent being, provoking numerous texts, including a particularly enervating[5] one by CS Lewis entirely devoted to its discussion – might actually prove that God does exist. Only a He could foresee the development of the medical profession and create the otherwise pointless entity of abdominal pain. So the next time the patient can't be bothered with your questions and just wants you to make the pain go away, you can inform them that the only reason they have the pain is so that they can tell you all about it.[6]

Acute abdominal pain

We're going to ignore this. If we think of this tome as some sort of preparation for medical exams (and I implore you not to ...), then there is no way that you should ever come across acute abdominal pain in such a situation. Imagine having 15 ham-fisted medical students karate-chopping *your* ruptured appendix. Alternatively, if we see it as a preparation for our lives as a physician (ditto ...), then dealing with the acute abdomen comes down to learning one phrase.

'Sounds surgical to me.'

It is not generally recognised by the public that the question uppermost in the mind of the doctor seeing them on arrival in Accident and Emergency is not 'What is the diagnosis?' but 'Who am I gonna get to look after this patient?' In the past, many hospitals left this decision to the porter manning the reception desk. Simple criteria sufficed so the surgical resident would answer his bedside phone at 3a.m. to hear the brief instruction 'abdo pain, Doc' or 'condition of lower body, Doc', while the medical SHO would get just about everything else. In these more enlightened days, the task of deciding who sees what is undertaken by the Accident and Emergency doctors. Any suggestion that this has improved things could only come from a very stupid person or a surgeon (no relation) – since easing the life of the latter seems to be its only function. It works like this:

Any attempt by Accident and Emergency staff to get a surgeon to see a patient, let alone take over their care, meets with the classical three-phase response of:

1 *unanswered page ... followed by*
2 *page answered by colleague or minion who says that the paged guy is very busy (presumably answering the page of this guy to say how busy he is) ... followed eventually by*

---

[5] Amazing word. Means exactly the opposite of what it appears to.
[6] A flaw in this argument exists with toothache. This might also be viewed as a useless miserableness except to let you know that you need to see the dentist. But if an all-powerful, all-bounteous God had foreseen the existence of dentists, surely he'd have done something about it?

3   *the pagee himself phoning to say he's just about to go into theatre* (to do what? – they've successfully avoided having contact either with or about anything resembling a patient all day), while in the background we hear this year's classical sound bite being interrupted by a referee's whistle.

So, since they can't have patients hanging around the Casualty corridor all night, the Accident and Emergency team follow the line of least resistance and bring all patients in under the medical banner, knowing that medical middle-management doctors will be too busy to check out their story. Thus cholecystitis gets brought in under the medics to 'exclude myocardial infarction'. It's a frequent feature of a medical post-receiving ward round to ask a patient when their chest pain started, only to be told 'What chest pain? It was down here, nearer my groin!'

Accident and Emergency rationalisation can be quite imaginative. Seventy-year-old women who fall and fracture a femur are 'off their feet', head injuries are 'query seizures?', and people who get hit by a baseball bat are 'people who got hit by a baseball bat probably because they fell out with someone because their diabetes is unstable'.

So, in a desperate attempt to turn the tide, I vote that we physicians learn nothing at all about acute abdominal pain, though when it does turn out to be the pesky 'diabetic ketoacidosis presenting as abdominal pain', let's hope the surgeons haven't used the same ploy and avoided learning any medicine – rather a forlorn hope since it would fly in the face of the past 100 years.

Chronic ('abdominal') pain

Heartburn

Burning over the heart. What could be simpler? Sometimes an acid taste in the back of the mouth (this does not equal 'water brash'). Sometimes increased burping.[7] Made worse by lying down (makes sense) or its being around 8.22p.m. as one is sitting watching the TV after a big meal. Also made worse by some idiosyncratic foods. Chocolate, fats, peppermint,[8] alcohol – theoretically because they relax the lower oesophageal sphincter,[9] which is paid to keep the gastric juice out of the gullet. My own *bêtes noires* are pork pies and Sauvignon Blanc white wine, but not Chardonnay. The New Zealand versions of sav blanc seem to be

---

[7] **Glib Explanation No. 2**. Even though saliva is slightly acidic, it's less so than the acid (hydrochloric – but I only mention this in case your future includes an important TV quiz show) in the stomach. So if you've got acid irritating your gullet, you swallow more saliva in an attempt to combat it (this isn't something you do deliberately – any more than you deliberately overbreathe to combat the acidosis in ketoacidosis). Swallow saliva, swallow air. This mounts up and results in burping ('flatulence' – not to be confused with 'flatus' unless you're writing comic scripts). Excessive burping as a symptom in isolation is simply a manifestation of air swallowing in someone who likes to annoy doctors. This can be 'cured' by having the patient bite a pen between their teeth. Admittedly a short-term remedy, but it proves the point.

[8] A popular flavouring for antacid remedies such as Gaviscon®, Maalox®, etc., peppermint is supposed to help release 'postprandial pressure' by facilitating burping. A dubious benefit that is almost certainly overshadowed by its increasing gastro-oesophageal reflux itself. I'd stick to aniseed (and so tasty!).

[9] The traditional name 'cardiac sphincter' has apparently been dropped, perhaps having caused confusion with affectionate terms for consultant colleagues during telephone conversations.

particularly toxic, though it is more likely that suggesting a change from Sancerre to Burgundy might impress the right sort of client in your future years.

As mentioned earlier, the pain can sometimes take on a tight severity, perhaps associated with oesophageal spasm, similar to that of ischaemic heart disease – and night-time episodes accompanied by a cold sweat can cause diagnostic difficulties in either direction.[10]

Troublesome nocturnal pain can often be improved by raising the head of the bed and decreasing regurgitation. The simple manoeuvre of using extra pillows does not succeed in the same way as elevating the entire head of the bed, e.g. with a good book or two. Two copies of this one would make an ideal package, and much cheaper than omeprazole for the rest of your life.

Dyspepsia/indigestion

This used to be much more interesting as a symptom. We'd take great care to elicit whether pains were worse before eating (duodenal ulcer), after eating (gastric ulcer) or during the night (duodenal), and what other things eased or exacerbated the discomfort. Unfortunately, this has all rather gone out the window because (a) it was all tosh, (b) nobody can be bothered to spend that much time taking a history and (c) the ubiquitous availability of upper gastrointestinal endoscopy means that if there is any mention of 'indigestion' (and, let's face it, we don't even bother to find out what is meant by that) we put the patient down for one. I suppose that's part of the appeal of a good 'service' from the gastroenterologists – it makes up for our slackness as history takers and clinicians. So just tell all patients to stop taking the anti-inflammatories (that they shouldn't be taking anyway for vague aches and pains), and if it doesn't go away we'll get those nice gastrointestinal people to put down a telescope/camera thingy.[11]

Vomiting

Oh, all right, there are upper gastrointestinal symptoms other than pain. There's vomiting. A tremendously non-specific symptom. Anything from psychogenic to 'dietary indiscretion'[12] – and we've mentioned earlier its association with any severe pain. Timing, precipitants and the nature of the vomitus itself are all important – and as an example we'll look at the acute vomiting scenario that most often involves the general physician. Haematemesis. Or, more correctly, 'query haematemesis' or '?haematemesis'.

As part of their 'no patients please, we're surgeons' policy, most hospitals have their haematemesis cases looked after by the medics. This means that any patient who presents with vomiting (which, barring infection, might otherwise suggest some acute surgical abdominal problem as the first option) is immediately told

---

[10] I remember one particular post-receiving patient who had tight pain throughout the night – accompanied by sweating but otherwise very well. He'd forgotten his omeprazole the previous two days. I was in a particularly confident position to reassure him, having had a very similar night for very similar reasons ... All his cardiac enzyme results came back *off the scale* ...

[11] A gastrointestinal colleague has indignantly pointed out that the discovery of *Helicobacter pylori* has *totally* changed all this. First they do a breath test, eradicate any *Helicobacter*, and when that doesn't help ... *then* they put down the telescope/camera thingy.

[12] This is the accepted euphemism for behaving like a two-year-old and eating/drinking everything you can lay your hands on. The acronym 'DI' is useful in the standard scenario of a curry followed by 12 pints of lager followed by the infamous desire for a kebab, where the sufferer may clearly express the view that they are 'wanting to DI'.

that they have been vomiting 'altered blood, haven't they?' and referred to the physicians as 'query haematemesis'. By the time you come to take the history, these patients will have been trained by Accident and Emergency staff (if this was not already their own opinion) to consider anything in their vomitus not immediately recognisable as a piece of Kentucky Fried Chicken to be altered blood. The classic example of this is the 'coffee-grounds' description so beloved of said Accident and Emergency staff. Anyone who will admit to this appearance in their vomitus – even if they've had nothing to eat all day but finely-ground coffee beans – will be assured that this is blood. For good measure, an FOB-type test may be performed (as vomitus will pretty much always show up 'positive for blood'). The fact that lots of vomiting people will eventually bring up some dark-bile-mixture stuff which could easily be termed coffee grounds is conveniently ignored.

To combat this ploy, one must take a detailed history of the vomiting – with particular regard to the sequence of events. And here we're moving into one of those tricky areas. One of the times when we're almost verging on the 'inter-rogation' of the patient like a witness at a trial. Nasty, evil doctors. Remember, everybody knows that nobody could possibly want to come into hospital unneces-sarily. This is of course true – except for the small number of people who want to come into hospital unnecessarily. We've discussed possible reasons for this, but here it's worth noting that among the main groups at risk of haematemesis are patients with alcohol problems. They may have many reasons why a stay in hospital might suit them, or indeed be required for them, but the easiest channel for them might be to ... embellish a story to suggest haematemesis. This does not mean for a moment that they are not worthy of care (and it is the fear of accusations of holding such views that can prevent doctors from stating things which they believe to be true), but that care does not include an incorrect diagnosis (care rarely does) from a knee-jerk reaction. Close history taking might save any sort of patient from an unnecessary endoscopy.[13]

Sometimes it won't make sense.

'Just eaten a big meal when I started to vomit up lots of those café-grounds (sic)' – but the food all stays down ... presumably the coffee grounds sneak past it.

'Vomited lots and lots of food until it suddenly changed to altered blood' – which presumably had been lying there, waiting to alter before it made an appearance on its own – but only after they'd run out of food. This story might do better for simply vomiting stomach contents then getting down to duodenal/bile/ugly stuff.

Cynical Tip No. 9   If the patient volunteers the phrase 'coffee grounds' then this is because someone has suggested it to them. This may be at some previous occasion, or someone somewhere wants to persuade you that this is a haematemesis. This may be the patient him- or herself, or another prac-titioner. This does not mean that the patient has *not* had a haematemesis, but you should be aware of the distinction. Don't assume 'coffee grounds' = haematemesis.

---

[13] In our enforced rush to practise defensive medicine – an over-investigative approach in an attempt to ensure that no diagnosis, however unlikely, is missed – we tend to forget that the investigations themselves can cause harm, or at the very least discomfort and inconvenience.

Just taking people nice and easy through their story of what happened can give you a very good idea of ... what happened. Particularly if the story changes when they try to make it more sensible. Of course, we all have to change our story on occasions (though when you think about it, just when are those?) – but sometimes you have to admit to the feeling that someone is ... 'making it up'. Not the sort of thing I'm supposed to say. Everybody points out how stressful it is to be ill (it is), how stressful it is to be in hospital (it is – though arguably being in hospital makes being ill less stressful), how stressful it is to be asked questions (particularly by a doctor?!), and so people may keep changing their story for various reasons. I agree this is the case. But I think it is narrow-minded (in a politically correct and therefore generally considered broad-minded sort of way) to dismiss out of hand the simple explanation outlined in:

Heresy Tip No. 5 **You are most likely to keep changing your story if you do not have the truth to fall back on.**

It's true. Sometimes you can see it in people's eyes[14] when you ask questions about timing or details of symptoms. Or there may be pauses before answering each question – like someone in *Inspector Morse*. Rather than simply answering your question, they are first trying to remember what they've said earlier, and if it makes sense, and if it's compatible with what they are about to say ... and if they find they've said something that is clearly impossible they say 'Oh, I'm all confused ... all these questions ... '

The 'regular attender'[15] may give up very early on any façade that we have a normal doctor–patient relationship going on:

> *'What have you been feeling wrong, sir?'*
> *'Vomiting up blood.'*
> *'When did it start?'*
> *'Oh, I don't know.'*
> *'Well, when was it you first had the vomiting?'*
> *'Look ... how should I know? ... you're getting me confused with all these*
>   *questions ... '*

---

[14] Nothing to do with all that psychobabble of looking to the left side of your brain when you're trying to manufacture an answer rather than trying to remember it (supposedly whereupon you'll look to the right, or is it the other way round?). This is proper science we're talking here. They look ... *shifty* ...

[15] The UK equivalent of the oft-quoted Americanism 'GOMER' (**G**et **O**ut of **M**y **E**mergency **R**oom). Such patients are generally recognised by doctors, nurses, porters ... everybody ... as being keen on staying in hospital (despite the fact that 'no one would ever possibly ... etc ... ') and will turn up regularly at the A and E department with a story that – taken at face value – cries out for admission. In our increasingly 'litigious society' it is increasingly difficult to send such people home – and indeed there is always the human/medical rather than legal worry (it's difficult to ignore the boy who cries wolf if you're paid to be the official wolf catcher) that this time it could be for real. In an increasingly politically correct society, it is also difficult to mention their very existence without coming under a hail of self-righteous accusation.

Another (possible) indicator of insincerity may be disgust at having the questions asked 'all over again'. Review by the consultant or other senior is thus seen as some sort of imposition, whereas most ill people are only too happy to go through their story again and again until somebody gets it right.

Cynical Tip No. 10 Patients who resent going through their story again may lack confidence that it will be the same one.

You may have spotted a veritable barrage of Cynical Tips. There is a reason. It's unlikely you could ever be faced with a 'query haematemesis' in exam conditions, as one doesn't 'use' acutely unwell patients. Hence my sneaky introduction of a totally unwarranted distrust in patients' credibility at this particular point – as it should go a long way towards achieving the desired goal of having this book banned. Clearly I must be prevented from poisoning the minds of embryonic medics, and while Establishment Man can weed out some of the blasphemy at examination time, that possibility does not arise with haematemesis. They will therefore be obliged to nip such heresy in the bud.

However, this thought process fails to allow for one of the latest 'advances' in exam organisation.

Actors.

Playing the part of patients or their relatives.

This device has been popular for some years in the Ethics and Communication sections of the MRCP exam, where actors simulate bereaved relatives, or someone who's waiting for you to tell them that they've got cancer. It is rather disconcerting as an examiner watching a distressed spouse break down in tears for the seventh time that afternoon while some poor candidate has to try to console them in the growing knowledge that (a) they are only pretending and (b) whether they are consoled or not depends entirely on the actor's whim rather than on how well the candidate really does. Now that they are using actors to play actual patients giving a history, I feel someone ought to call a halt. Once any competent candidate has taken a story from one of these 'patients', the only answer to the question 'What's the diagnosis?' that would impress me is 'He's having us on. There's nothing wrong with him'.

What is the point of 'testing' a candidate such that he or she passes by saying that a perfectly healthy person has had an MI, or a haematemesis? You might as well pick a poker team full of people who always believe the other guy's bluff, referees who ask players politely if they were offside, or judges who believe a defendant is innocent until it's proven that ... (we'll leave that one) ...

And the actor has a huge role (hoorah!) in deciding how smoothly things go for the candidate. They can take a liking to them ... or not.[16] They can get fed up after the first two or three and start mucking about to make things more interesting. They might take exception because you're unravelling their lack of knowledge of their symptoms or illness. And their story might not make any sense ... because ... *they don't have the truth to fall back on* ...

---

[16] Will the over-achieving of pretty blondes in medical exams improve even further?

So maybe now they *will* give you a '?haematemesis' in the exam, and you can have fun dipping back and forward into their story, getting them to add the most unlikely extensions until it collapses like a house of cards, before announcing proudly to the examiner that 'this chancer is making the whole thing up'.

Then, as the patient is taken back down to the ward for the rest of their transfusion, you can take the time to work out a study programme for the resits. Two more tips on vomiting before we go.

Cynical Tip No. 11   A patient attending your gastroenterology clinic who is actively retching[17] and burping should be viewed with some suspicion.

Spelling Tip No. 1   One *t*.

Bowel habit (whatever that is)

Everybody's different. We were always taught that 'normal' frequency of bowel movements was anything from three times per day to once every three days – and even that probably underestimates normal variation. It's a change from the patient's own norm which is important (and, of course, the patient's own norm might be 'variable'). So if a 70-year-old man has moved his bowels every other day for $69\frac{5}{8}$ years, but three times per day for the past four months, it's worth looking into. Alternating diarrhoea/constipation might be particularly suspicious (though again this can be long-standing, as in irritable bowel syndrome). Generally constipated with occasional watery motions might suggest the 'spurious diarrhoea' of a[18] (sort-of partial) obstruction.

Now for the bad news. The consistency, texture – whatever you want to call it – of the stools is also very important. But if you thought patients were less helpful than they might have been with sputum, just wait till you try getting them to describe their stools. They'll admit to 'diarrhoea', but any qualifying inquiry simply makes them think you're crazy. They lose all sense of quantity, texture or even colour. Black sticky stuff (melaena[19]), dark runny stuff (infective, dietary indiscretion), runny stuff plus bits plus mucus (severe infective, colitis), blood-stained runny stuff (ditto), pale and bulky and floating (fat malabsorption) and green (late infective with dehydration) all become just 'diarrhoea', and that's as far as you get. I suppose the patient's got a point when it comes to one of our ingenious[20] enquiries – as to whether the stools are foul-smelling. Anything else sounds pathological to me.

Duration is also of huge importance. Infective diarrhoeal illnesses are among the most miserable things in the world. Many, such as *Campylobacter*, mimic ulcerative

---

[17] Vomiting without vomit. Referred to in Scotland as 'the dry boak'.

[18] I wonder if that should be *a* or *an*? Indeed, read that question out loud and maybe we have to change the *a*. Should have done it the other way round.

[19] You will not be surprised to learn that any diarrhoea darker than a snowman's will be termed 'melaena' by our favourite A and E staff members – for reasons which will by now be apparent. Real melaena is sticky and tarry, not just dark.

[20] Couldn't read my draft writing whether this was *ingenuous* or an ironic *ingenious*. Still not sure. In the past, I invariably used it ironically, but recently … yowza! … **altered vowel habit!**

colitis or Crohn's disease with systemic upset, profuse diarrhoea – potentially bloody, slimy – even with similar endoscopic appearances. But they don't tend to last more than a week, after which inflammatory bowel disease becomes more likely. And, of course, duration of symptoms is always something that even the vaguest of patients should be able to help you with …

Jaundice

Doc: 'So what's been the problem?'
Patient: 'The jandees.'[21]
Doc: 'The jandees?'
Patient: 'Aye, the jandees. The yellow jandees.'
Doc: 'And how long have ye had it … them?'[22]
Patient: 'Oh, for quite a wee while now.'
Doc: 'And how long's that?'
Patient: 'Oh, quite a while.'
Doc: 'But how long's "quite a while"?'
Patient: 'Ages.'
Doc: 'But how long's "ages"?'
Patient: 'Quite a while.'
Doc: 'But how long is that? Two days?'
Patient: 'Naw. More than two days.'
Doc: 'Two months?'
Patient: 'Naw. Not as much as two months.'
Doc: 'So … more than two days, less than two months … a month maybe?'
Patient: 'Aye – about that.'
Doc: 'So you've had them about a month?'
Patient: 'Had what?'
Doc: 'THE JANDEES!'
Patient: 'Aw, the jandees … aye, they've been for quite a wee while now … '

The man in the street's attitude to jaundice is a bit of a puzzle. While a number of other symptoms that doctors treat with a dismissive (but carefully considered) grain of salt (tight-band-around-the-head-ache; boring pain under the left nipple,[23] fresh red blood at the end of defaecation, vertex headache, pains all over, piercing, lancinating pain through the left eyeball … or is that just me? …) strike fear into the heart of the layman, he'll often regard jaundice as hardly worth an incidental mention. Yet, other than the occasional benign virus or gallstone (surgical!!), jaundice is usually a sign that something is up – including, more often than one would like, the game.

Jaundice (essentially raised bilirubin levels in the blood causing pigmentation of the tissues) is a 'nice' exam scenario, since it splits into three distinct types which can often be pinpointed by focused questioning.

1 *Haemolytic jaundice* – caused by breakdown of red blood cells in the blood with release of their haemoglobin and breakdown pigment bilirubin.

---

[21] Jandees = jaundice in Scottish (Glasgow) parlance.
[22] … and of course, is (are) plural.
[23] The official title of which – 'atypical left submammary chest pain' – goes very little way towards convincing anxious sufferers that the medical practitioner isn't making it up as he goes along.

2 *Hepatitic jaundice* – caused by damage to the liver cells with release of bilirubin which has been mopped up by the liver and is being conjugated in the cells.

3 *Obstructive jaundice* – results when the outflow of bile into the duodenum is interrupted, and with no way out, there is eventual leakage of bilirubin into the blood. Classically due to, for example, a gallstone blocking the bile duct, a similar pattern occurs with multiple blocking 'further up' of the tiny ducts in the liver – when the alternative term 'cholestatic jaundice' for some reason feels to me more appropriate.[24]

Amazingly, asking patients about their urine and (aaargh!) stools can pretty much pigeon-hole any jaundice. Here's how. Bilirubin is conjugated in the liver cells (making it, among other things, water soluble), then gets into the gut as part of bile oozing into the duodenum at the ampulla of Vater. Further down in the gut, it is converted to other pigments, including stercobilin (part of the reason why faeces are ... brown?)[25] and urobilinogen (which gets reabsorbed back into the blood as part of the enterohepatic circulation thingy, eventually making its way to the urine – hence name – where it is normally present in small quantities and, being more colourless/yellow, is part of the reason why urine is ... but you know the rest).

So:

If you've got *haemolytic jaundice*, you'll have extra bilirubin in the blood from lysed cells. This bilirubin ain't conjugated, so it ain't water soluble and doesn't get into the urine (it's all stuck on to albumin and is unfilterable) – so urine doesn't become red/dark.[26] You do make excess urobilinogen from the bilirubin in the gut and so the urine has excess urobilinogen, making it ... *very* colourless/yellowish. Bowel motions are not interfered with – so no change there.

Hepatitic jaundice – some of the bilirubin coming from the cells will have been conjugated, so the urine will go a bit red/dark. Meanwhile, bilirubin pigment will still get through to the gut, and bowel movements will be largely unaltered. Similarly, urobilinogen will be made in the bowel and get to the urine as normal.

Obstructive jaundice – the bile/bilirubin/pigment stuff doesn't get through to the gut ... it spills over into the blood. It's conjugated so it helps to cause 'red' urine. But since it can't get through to the gut, there's no enterohepatic circulation so (a) there is no pigment in the faeces – stools become pale and (b) no urobilinogen is made – difficult to judge if the urine is less colourless/yellow than normal, but stix testing will show an abnormal absence of urobilinogen.

---

[24] Gastroenterologists are now more likely to divide jaundice into haemolytic, hepatic and post-hepatic – lumping cholestatic into the middle section. Further evidence of a move from how-to-diagnose-what's-wrong towards who-looks-after-this-patient? The only reason why cholestatic, which has the same findings as post-hepatic, would be lumped with hepatitic is because it is medical, not surgical.

[25] I have to admit it's all a bit hazy exactly which degradations take place where (where does stercobilinogen fit in?). Probably not mulled over enough at cocktail parties.

[26] Hence haemolytic jaundice was known by the Ancients as 'acholuric jaundice', since there was 'no bile' in the urine. This explanation assumes you know that *a* or *an* from the Greek ... '*a*' means 'absence of', 'not' or 'without', as in *a*plastic anaemia ... or indeed *an*aemia ... It should, of course, be used only where the rest of the word is also derived from ancient Greek, any other use being intrinsically amoral.

So, again:

- normal urine, normal stools – haemolytic.
- dark urine, normal stools – hepatitic.
- dark urine, pale stools – obstructive (cholestatic).

We'll make no mention of 'mixed pictures', as that would ruin a good story.

Obstructive jaundice is also reputed to cause itching more than the others, as well as a greenish tinge (I've absolutely no idea whether this has anything to do with biliverdin, an intermediate breakdown product) – 'the green jandees'.[27]

Patients with jaundice should be asked about their alcohol intake, but also about viral symptoms, recent contacts, immunisations, blood transfusions, foreign travel, drug use (legal and otherwise) ... and it's OK if you wear gloves while taking blood. Whether you feel obliged to question them about their sexual preferences may depend on how fruitful other lines of enquiry have been.

Weight

This is hugely important when assessing patients. A story of genuine weight loss turns the feeblest of histories into a worrying one. Yet the traditional meticulous documentation by nursing staff of the weight of every patient admitted to hospital is in many places falling by the wayside. It seems that nurses are too busy with the 'nursing process', asking patients about symptoms, drugs, allergies (things that PRHOs used to do when they were JHOs,[28] but they are now themselves too busy phoning up labs and painting their nails), which side they dress on[29] and their preferred flavour of marmalade. Even patients admitted because of weight loss appear to have this investigation omitted! So if your patient says they've lost two stones in six months and you discover they were in hospital six months ago, don't expect the case notes to confirm the details. They won't. Make it one of your quests to right this wrong.

Examination

General inspection includes looking for the jandees (best in the sclerae and, oddly, the skin of the abdomen) and evidence of weight loss. Chronic liver disease can cause easy bruising, a thin veined appearance to the skin (e.g. of the face – 'paper-money skin') and the famous 'spider naevi'. These little inflamed/expanded capillaries/venules/arterioles probably do look a bit like little red spiders, if such things exist (though probably they more closely resemble the inside of a red nutmeg). For some inexplicable reason, they occur anywhere on the skin in the

---

[27] It's not known whether the monks and nuns of the Carthusian Order near Grenoble were making a veiled reference (as nuns do) to the different hues of jaundice when they decided on colours for their Chartreuse liqueur. The naming of one of the stronger pipe tobaccos after the founder of the Order (St Bruno) might lend further weight to the suggestion of a rather debauched lifestyle among the Orders of the day (is this what was meant by the 'dissolution of the monasteries'?).

[28] *See* Chapter 10 on Haematology.

[29] *See* Appendix 1.

drainage area of the superior vena cava (basically any part of the body above the nipple). Three to four are allowed as a variant of normal.[30]

Hands again offer finger clubbing as a talking point − occurring in inflammatory bowel disease (possibly Crohn's disease more often than ulcerative colitis) and cirrhosis of the liver. Chronic liver disease throws up an absolute cornucopia of peripheral manifestations. As well as exhibiting clubbing, the nails may be whiter than normal (leukonychia), while the palms may be red around the ulnar border and base (palmar erythema − also seen in pregnancy, rheumatoid arthritis and, apparently, thyrotoxicosis). Dupuytren's contracture[31] may be associated with liver disease or the likely accompanying alcohol habit. Any progression of the disease to hepatic encephalopathy (an early indication of which may be a tendency to invert the diurnal rhythm − sleeping during the day with night-time wakefulness[32]) may be accompanied by the 'flapping' asterixis mentioned with CO_2 retention, and the dyspraxic inability to draw a six-pointed star.[33] An advance on this assessment may be the 'Trail Test', in which the patient has to connect numbers randomly spread on a piece of paper. This is usefully quantitative, as the measured time can be used to monitor progress more accurately than 'good star' vs. 'bad star'.

'Examine the abdomen'

OK − there was an awful lot of stuff to look for in the hands. So, as we've touched on before, if you are asked in the exam to 'examine the abdomen', do you look at the hands? And the answer, again, is 'yes − but don't take all day'. You can tag it on to the end of that nasty little introducing-yourself-to-the-patient bit. Ooops. Did I say 'nasty'? This farrago has developed over the years from a brief 'OK-if-I-examine-you?' exchange − often at the level of body language − to an overly effusive welcome, introduction and brief-potted-personal-history ritual which suggests that you may wish not so much to examine the patient's hand as to ask for that of his daughter in marriage.

This ritual is increasingly accompanied by an exchange of first names (not a real exchange − you offer yours, but the patient's is in the case sheets, on your list,

---

[30] As a rule of thumb, answer any question along the lines 'What is generally accepted as within normal?' with *'three or four'*. It works for almost everything − spiders, cm of JVP, beats of clonus, inches of chest expansion … but not for thumbs themselves.

[31] This thickening of the palmar aponeurosis causes flexion contractures most often affecting the ring finger, then the pinkie in liver disease. In diabetes, it more often affects the middle finger as second choice.

[32] As with the St Bruno reference, the similarity to the lifestyle of a medical student is probably coincidental.

[33] To me, this has always appeared an unfair challenge for the unsuspecting patient − who has probably not contemplated drawing a six-pointed star since the age of twelve. It is normal to first demonstrate exactly what is required − though this may further disadvantage the patient by suggesting that *your* technique for performing this useless task (draw overlapping triangles? … think overlapping triangles? … draw at random? …) is perforce the one that the patient should adopt. And he hasn't been practising for years like you have (yes − you have! Imagine the potential embarrassment of a wizened 90-year-old alcoholic the colour of a bottle of either Chartreuse pausing briefly from his litre of vodka to draw a six-pointer which is manifestly more precise than your own …).

even up on the wall for everyone to see). This is an irritating practice which seems to have wormed its way from the habit of the 'caring profession'[34] of asking 'Jimmy' for his intimate details, seconds after he has arrived in the ward, as if they'd known him all his life (except then you'd know better than to ask him about such things). While an improvement on thinking of a patient as 'Bed Number 16',[35] this familiarity is unbecoming. A 67-year-old retired judge does not necessarily wish to be called 'Jimmy' by a whippersnapper of either sex just out of school. Nor may a 67-year-old retired plumber ... odd-job man ... or cardiologist. It may appear to add a 'human touch', but to me it smacks more of treating the patient as the inmate of a boarding-school. And the idea that giving the patient your own first name somehow helps ... doesn't. Giving anyone your first and not your second name is the opposite of an introduction. It keeps you apart from them – out of each other's life. The guy who serves you in McDonald's tells you his first name, not your doctor. The guy who gets you up from dinner to answer the phone so that he can try to sell you double-glazing tells you his first name. These people have no wish for the real connection that giving someone your second name implies – because it tells them who you are.[36]

And the badges would be a major embarrassment.

So, if you must introduce yourself, I suggest (from the deeply scientific stance of 'in my opinion'[37]) that you say your first and second name – that's a real introduction – with no plans to start calling the patient by their first name unless they request this ... or are eight years old.

So ... examine the abdomen. While 45° for JVPs, etc. was a bit arbitrary, it is genuinely helpful to follow the rules and get the patient fairly flat for abdominal examination. No matter how many times you've seen the consultant poke a diffident hand into a patient seated at their bedside with a cursory 'tummy OK?', this is a case of 'do as I say not as I do'. This is not a licence to put somebody with rampant left ventricular failure through the equivalent of being held under in the bathtub while you squelch their liver, but since any sitting up tenses the abdominal muscles and makes everything trickier, as flat as the patient feels comfortable is ideal.

The old surgical adage of preparing the abdomen for examination by having it 'bared from the nipples to the knees' is, of course, cruel (the clue was in the word 'surgical') and arguably illegal. Most patients would probably view it more gainly[38] to be entirely naked, and since most of us value an attempt to look cool over modesty regarding our private parts (how else do we explain mini-skirts, tight T-shirts and ... beaches?), this approach is worth avoiding. Other dilemmas remain, however. Do you go to the front of the bed to see if the abdomen is symmetrical, distended, yellow, 'moving normally with respiration' – whatever

---

[34] Nurses ... apparently ...

[35] Although this method does have an advantage in corridor discussions – when passers-by have no idea about whom you are talking – it would be disconcerting for the heart attack patient in bed 16 to undergo a sigmoidoscopy because the previous incumbent had 'altered bowel habit'.

[36] Heavy-breather phone callers don't tell you *their* surname ...

[37] The equivalent of 'C'-level recommendation in the old SIGN guidelines (A = according to randomised placebo-controlled studies; B = according to uncontrolled studies; C = according to a bunch of guys sitting round a table, or indeed one of their grannies who knows about such things ...).

[38] An attempt to accentuate the positive of a word we more usually see in the negative. I admit not up to PG Wodehouse's description of an unhappy character as 'far from being gruntled'.

that means? Answer. Yes. Nobody does it in real life, but it is the best way to assess most of these things. But don't knock over the examiner (or nurse) while getting there.

Palpation

Yeah. Sit down. Or kneel, if necessary. I am increasingly perplexed by the recent changes in the working lives of junior doctors. Among these is the way they sit when I think they should stand (giving case presentations at hospital meetings, listening to hearts, when I come into the room ...), but stand at times when one would traditionally sit (having lunch ... or other drinks) — including examining the abdomen. Kneeling when no seat is available may appear rather flamboyant, but it makes sense — as long as you don't try to demonstrate an obese spleen from an impossible angle.

Have I talked about sitting on the patient's bed yet? I must admit a tendency to sit on the patient's bed when taking their story. This is fairly near the foot of the bed, having checked with the patient that this is OK and that there's no unsuspecting shinbone under my chosen spot. This also tends to be on post-receiving ('post-take', 'post-waiting') ward rounds where the patient has a story to tell and there doesn't tend to be a handy chair at every bedside. To me, sitting on the edge of the bed is superior to standing (ironically enough). If a chair is available, I'll use it ... though I sometimes have to wonder if my tendency to sit on the arm of such an appliance — or at least slightly sideways — is simply affectation. For some reason I just don't like setting myself in any sort of formal position. As a registrar, I used to upset clinic nurses the first moment I walked in — immediately changing all the furniture round so that I wasn't sitting across a desk from the patient, which seemed so confrontational. Nowadays most clinic rooms are laid out such that a more 'friendly angle' is available as the norm.[39]

However ... although the taking of a history while seated on the bed is probably acceptable, examination of the patient — even of the hands — doesn't really work.[40]

Anyway:

- *Do* sit or kneel down when examining the abdomen.
- *Do* ask the patient if they're tender anywhere.
- *Do* do that first superficial all-over palpation (no digging in!) thing to confirm this (it's not that we don't trust patients, but ... oh, forgot ...).

---

[39] It would be pretentious (a word I've chosen — to leave the possibility in the mind of the reader that the claim may be true — in place of the more accurate phrase 'absolute tosh') to claim I'd single-handedly revolutionised such practices. Nevertheless, I do remember persistently being 'cautioned' by my erstwhile professor to put on my white coat. Nowadays nobody seems to wear these (hoorah!), though the legions of nubile young JHOs in T-shirts which flaunt their perfect belly-buttons (or umbilici, as the professor would have called them) whenever they lean over to pick up a pen (dropped by whom?) have perhaps taken it a bit too far.

[40] There are two occasions when we legitimately rest on the bed. One is while performing 'confrontational examination of the visual fields' (which, despite my previous rants, in no way involves accusing the patient of deliberately turning a blind eye), and the other is during the exquisitely awkward manoeuvre of assessing chest expansion from the back — where otherwise your left knee will almost certainly end up wedged somewhere between the pillow and either the patient's or your own axilla (by this time you will not realise which).

- *Do* glance at the patient's face while doing this (in case they are stoically suffering excruciating pains in silence so as not to offend) but ...
- *Don't* overdo this and *not* glance at the abdomen itself (among other things, you don't want to accidentally put your hand somewhere inappropriate ...).
- *Do* assess any odd masses before moving on to individual organs ...
- *Do* have a quick feel (but don't call it that) for a lymph node in the supraclavicular fossae. A node in the left is a pointer to carcinoma in the upper abdomen, classically gastric. Interestingly, two separate ancients are immortalised in this finding. If you have *Virchow's ('Virkov's') node*, then that's *Troisier's sign*.

Liver

- *Do* get the patient to breathe in and out (it will surprise them that this is allowed, then surprise you that you have to teach them how. Their natural tendency is to breathe in at entirely the wrong moment).
- *Do* confirm that any liver edge isn't just 'pushed down' by emphysema. Percuss for the position of the top edge of the liver. There will be a book somewhere which will tell you where this should be. I could of course save every reader from having to go and find and look up such a book by stating the answer here ... but then *I'd* have to go and find and look up such a book, and it seems easier (from where I'm sitting) to leave it up to yous.[41]
- *Do* assess the liver edge (smooth/non-smooth, hard/firm/not, tender/not) and the *surface* (different thing) of the liver (smooth, not smooth, lumpy, very lumpy, craggy ...) – don't just say it's there.
- *Do* know how wide your fingerbreadths are.
- *Do* remember that funny bit medially where you think you can feel a liver edge but you can't really (or is that just me? ...). Nobody has satisfactorily explained this phenomenon to me – the fascial lines in the rectus abdominis (as in 'six-pack' effect) just don't convince me that they should feel like that. To me the clue to dismiss the finding is that the 'edge' suddenly disappears as I move laterally (while there can occur a Riedel's lobe or other expansion of the medial lobe of the liver, this is on the rare side).
- *Do* remember that established cirrhosis usually gives you a small impalpable liver – so don't panic when all the peripheral signs are there, but you can't feel a liver edge.

Spleen

- *Do* start in the right iliac fossa and move diagonally across (or vice versa). It *is* very rare for the spleen to enlarge that far, but just such novelties will jump the queue into exams.[42]

---

[41] A Scotticism of impeccable logic, since the absence of a plural 'yous' in English yields no great advantage to man nor beast nor language, while leaving open numerous opportunities for ambiguity.

[42] Hence the old adage 'common things occur commonly, but rare things aren't that rare ...', to which can be added '... especially in exams'.

- *Do* get the patient after the first palpation to lean on their right side for further palpation under the left ribs with hugely deep breathing (... by the patient, that is ...).
- *Don't* go back again at this point to the right iliac fossa.
- *Do* get the patient to cough while doing this palpation just to bring the spleen down that bit further (after all, everybody keeps telling us *ad nauseam* that the spleen can double its size and still not be palpable, so take any extra chance you can).
- If the above all fail, *do* percuss over the lowest left rib spaces antero-laterally (Traube's area) with the patient lying on their back. This should normally be resonant/tympanitic (supposedly because of the gastric bubble, though I blame the lungs – Traube was originally looking to diagnose pleural effusions), but with an enlarged spleen becomes dull – giving you a hint to go back and try again.

Kidneys

- *Do* get the patient to lie back flat again after you've got your hands into position.
- *Do* remember that they move on respiration (not a lot ...).
- *Do* remember that the lower pole of the right kidney may be palpable in a normal slim person.
- *Do* remember that there are two of them.

Do remember the ways to tell an enlarged left kidney from a spleen – even though you think there is no reason at all for anybody to ever get them mixed up[43] (we all think that ... and we all do). In the absence of anything else exciting, this is the only 'abdominal question' that any of us examiners is able to think of. Essentially, it's a collection of different ways (except No. 1) of saying that the spleen and the kidney are nowhere near each other.

1 The spleen may have a notch (yeah – three times in 25 years, and I suspect the third case was the first one back again 20 years later).
2 The spleen enlarges towards the right iliac fossa while the kidney enlarges ... up-and-down (doh! ...).
3 You can't get above a spleen (tucked up behind the ribs), but you can get above a kidney (i.e. it's retro-peritoneal).
4 You can get a 'band of resonance' (?transverse colon) over the kidney (i.e. it's retro-peritoneal).
5 The spleen moves more on respiration than the kidney (i.e. the latter is retro-peritoneal).
6 The kidney can be 'balloted' between both hands (i.e. it's retro ...).
7 Essentially exactly the same as (6) – but included as it's my personal favourite ... once you get a kidney between your two hands (i.e. it's ...) you can hold it there while getting the patient to take a deep breath in/out ... and then you release your fingers a tad and the kidney squelches up between your fingers ... yowzah!

---

[43] On first encountering this list, I thought 'might as well have a protocol for telling an eyeball from a nose' ... there probably is one for trauma plastic surgeons ...

Auscultation

Auscultation of the abdomen usually takes patients by surprise, but has four principal functions.

1 It covers up the times you automatically reach for your stethoscope when about to undertake the unfamiliar task of examining the abdomen. Make sure that you do not re-lose credibility by asking the patient to breathe in and out through their mouth while you listen.
2 You can listen for the rare bruit over a hepatoma (while gritting your hen's teeth).
3 You should listen for renal artery bruits in anyone with problematic hypertension. You press the bell of the stethoscope fairly firmly on to the abdomen just lateral to the umbilicus and listen intently for a murmur which sounds like an aortic ejection systolic murmur (if you don't know what that sounds like, stop reading this book immediately and go and see some patients). Its presence suggests renal artery stenosis – which is a pretty cool diagnosis to make clinically.
4 In some patients with dubious severe abdominal tenderness, performing the same manoeuvre as in (3) will magically elicit no pain whatsoever. This is not an unwarranted assault, as listening for bowel sounds is a mandatory part of examination in abdominal pain with tenderness (indeed, I bet some of you thought *that* was number (4) – but it's not, as that would be *surgical!*).

Addendum
(Have just performed a 'find ascites' on the edit menu and the word cannot be found in the document. It appears I have omitted to mention ascites anywhere in this book! An unforgivable omission, as this should be searched for at some stage in abdominal examination, even if not suggested by any general distension. The usual technique for finding ascites is slightly more tricky than dragging a menu and clicking.)

Shifting dullness/resonance
The abdomen is lightly percussed from the midline towards each flank in turn. The pleximeter finger is held vertically down the midline and worked across. The note *will* eventually change from tympanitic to dull at some stage. I suggest going all the way down to the flank – then, once you realise what dullness is, work your way back up again, defining where the note changes. This should be done on both sides and the two points marked gently with a ballpoint pen (having obtained the patient's informed consent[44]). The patient is then gently manoeuvred on to one side or the other and allowed to 'settle' (I usually get them on to their right side and use this opportunity to search for the spleen in this position – this saves them one more manoeuvre). The percussion is repeated, and if ascites is present the dullness on the dependent side moves up ('shifting resonance') and that on the upper side disappears ('shifting dullness').

Testing for 'fluid thrill' backs up the above proper test with a bit of fun. The examiner gets the examiner to help by placing the hilt of his hand along the

---

[44] Nowadays this probably requires you to tell the patient of all the inherent dangers and side-effects of having ballpoint pen markings on their abdomen. It could, after all, start them on the slippery slope to tattoo addiction.

midline of the patient's abdomen. This stops a 'fat thrill' through the adipose tissue. The examiner (i.e. the examiner, not the examiner) then places the flat of one hand against one flank (the patient's, not either examiner's) and 'flicks' the other flank with a finger (if there's any left, and being careful not to call it a 'flinger') as if knocking a wasp off a piece of gingerbread. If ascites is present the flick may be transmitted through the fluid to the receiving hand – but don't bet on it.

The nether regions

Do examine for inguinal lymphadenopathy.

Do examine the testicles (if appropriate ... and do ask ...) in a real-life patient – but simply mention the necessity for this in an exam (in the first instance).

Don't do a rectal examination in an exam. Again, mention its importance. In real life it is often difficult to decide whether rectal examination is necessary ... appropriate ... justifiable. I suppose it's a sign that we do indeed have sensitivity to a patient's feelings that we always think twice before performing a rectal (when you think about it – in among all the other stuff you do, it really isn't any major problem for the doctor). Clear-cut indications make it an easy decision. As does the simple help that the patient is attending with a gastrointestinal complaint – their expectations already doing the groundwork preparation for you to introduce this concept as a necessity. But if the patient has, for example, come up to the rheumatology clinic about their aching joints (where it often comes as a surprise to them that you ask them to take off their jacket) and you've found an unexplained iron deficiency with a minimum of bowel upset, it's a difficult subject to bring up.

I suppose what we do is weigh up the mutual embarrassment of a not clearly necessary rectal examination against the potential 'embarrassment' and other consequences of an unperformed rectal examination which turned out to be necessary after all.

Don't do internal examinations on women unless you're a gynaecologist or a GP. And if you're a GP, whatye doin' readin' a book?

Don't bother examining the hernial orifices (hurrah!) in a medical patient. Hernias (herniae?) are hugely surgical and, more importantly, chronic. So unless the surgeons can get their pals in Accident and Emergency to take over the vetting of referrals to outpatient clinics and pretend that all herniae (hernias) are caused by underlying thyroid disease until proven otherwise, we can thankfully leave the finger-poke-plus-cough procedure to the general surgeons[45] and sports medicine specialists.[46]

There is one problem here regarding the changing format of university exams. My own medical school, having been outed in *The Observer*'s investigation into

---

[45] Always a favourite when showing doctors assessing a line of fresh-faced army recruits. As if the discovery of a hernia so small it requires this examination to find it would ever stop your country's leaders from sacrificing the rest of your body to achieve its aims.

[46] Though the vogue for professional footballers and other sportspersons having operations to 'repair a small hernia' seems to be abating. Training methods may have improved, nomenclature may have changed (let's face it, a 'hernia' ain't exactly macho), but my bet is that sportsmen or their financial advisers have reviewed some statistics showing the decreased incidence of 'groin strain' (not requiring expensive surgery in a private clinic/hospital) coinciding with an increase in 'minor hernia' (opposite of 'ditto').

such establishments as being one of the three *best* in the United Kingdom, immediately decided that it would have to change everything. As well as introducing problem-based learning (PBL[47]) and other innovative teaching methods, a single long case has become the focus of the Finals. Students turn up for this unaware whether the case is medical, surgical, gynaecological or indeed psychiatric. The idea is that, since they don't know, they will be equally well prepared in all subjects, so testing one will essentially test them all.

The potential here for 'playing the odds' does seem enormous. It is reminiscent of the arguably apocryphal story of a European country, which we shall not identify, in which the medical schools are so large that examining all candidates in their Finals would be a logistical nightmare. Students therefore formed into groups of ten, from which one would be chosen at random to decide the fate of all of his or her colleagues. Not so daft as it seems. As the years of their course went by, students congregated into groups that would tend to contain ten students of a similar ability. The top guys in the year would obviously join together in one group so that any one of them would reflect their general ability, the second-best would also clump together, and so on. It sort of works.

Except.

Say one absolutely appalling student is also absolutely appallingly rich. Say he offers a bunch of smart types 100 000 Euros (oops − almost said 1 000 000 000 *lire* there ...) each to let him join their group? There's only a one-in-ten chance that this appalling student will be randomly picked to sit the exam (and even then he might pass) ... so the odds are quite good ... and it is an awful lot of money ...

However, back to the single long case.[48] Picking which subjects to study has always been the prerogative of the ... discerning student, so the lottery aspect does seem to fall short of criminal. One other fallout from the single case is an increasingly eccentric pairing of examiners. It has always been 'good form' for a Finals examiner to avoid close questioning in his own specialty, as it is difficult to judge competence (a diabetologist, for instance, may take for granted intimate knowledge of new insulin preparations that a cardiologist may never have heard of − assuming that they've heard of insulin), as it is the *general* medical knowledge of a *general* physician which is the gold standard. The current system takes this to new heights, and your history taking and examination of a 25-year-old man with paranoid schizophrenia might well be assessed by a gynaecologist and a colorectal surgeon. And if you don't examine the inguinal hernial orifices, you could be in trouble ...

Which leads obliquely to my final tip.

Do have a chaperone with you whenever possible ... for everyone's sake.

---

[47] PBL − you know the thing. A group of 8−10 students are given a scenario and they all go their separate ways to study its different aspects. They come back together to share their knowledge and insights. Designed to better imprint learning as well as training students to fend for themselves, unfortunately it can result in groups slipping into their own formulaic pattern. Individuals persist in doing the bit they're best at. In the scenario of young girl falling off bike, Jamie may not know how to tell if she's broken any bones, but will know how her islets of Langerhans cells will respond (and indeed how they will respond to pneumonia, myocardial infarction and meals-on-wheels). Meantime Jacqi will know how to assess for injury to the handle-bars ...

[48] No longer called the long case for reasons we needn't discuss here − though it is made longer by the candidate's legitimately running off in the middle of it to look up medical textbooks (no one has yet offered the examiners this facility).

5

Neurology

Neurologists differ from the rest of us. Even their motto is different. Instead of *Primum non Nocere* ('first do no harm') they have *Primum Nihil Facere* ('first do no ... thing'). But at least they compensate by having extra mottoes ... *Secundum Nihil Facere ... Tertium Nihil Facere ...*

You see, neurologists don't actually do anything – or at least don't actually treat anything. This first came to my attention in the dog-eat-dog world of clinical pharmacology when my boss was searching for a niche – to get away from the ubiquitous cardiovascular pharmacology that everyone pursued.

'Epilepsy is the way ahead,' he decided.

'Don't the neurologists look after that?'

He looked at me gravely ... 'How old are you, exactly? ... '

So I thought about it. He was right. Neurologists didn't really look after epilepsy. They just diagnosed it and let the patients attend their clinic once every year or so for a pat on the back. So I considered other 'neurological' conditions. Strokes were looked after by 'stroke experts' (cardiovascular or geriatric), Parkinson's disease by geriatricians,[1] migraine by GPs ... and I realised – neurologists didn't treat *anything*. They were simply diagnosticians. They could diagnose things precisely but they didn't try to make them better. So they filled up their clinics with interesting diseases like multiple sclerosis and motor neurone disease which they could diagnose, but couldn't do anything about.

This is why, as a GP, you send a letter to a cardiologist saying that you think this patient has angina, and they see the patient and write back ...

> I think you're right. Start aspirin 75 mg daily and atenolol at 25 mg per day, increasing the dose if no better – then add in a nitrate if beta-blocked and pulse already down around 60. I'll organise an ETT and an angio then we'll ... etc ...

But if you write asking a neurologist for an opinion on someone whom you think has MS, they see the patient and write back ...

> I think you're right.
> Regards,
>   J Smith, Neurologist ... etc ....

Recently, however, things have gone a bit weird for them. *Treatments* have appeared for some of their pet diseases. Fortunately, most are 'controversial'. Patient groups have to knock down the doors of Parliament in order to obtain

---

[1] Non-PC term (*see* Chapter 7 on Gerontology).

interferon for their multiple sclerosis, riluzole for their motor neurone disease or donepezil for their mother's Alzheimer's disease. Presumably this is all a co-incidence, and neurological drugs just happen to be ones with doubtful benefits. It seems unlikely that neurologists are so entrenched in their no-treatment position that they would actively block the prospect of making people better ...

Meanwhile, more neurologists than before are taking an interest in treating the bread-and-butter diseases such as epilepsy and parkinsonism. This has been accompanied by unprecedented advances in drug therapy – a chicken-and-egg scenario where cynics might suggest that the advances embarrassed the neurologists into getting involved in treating patients, rather than their actually making the advances. Whatever the impetus, the afore-mentioned clinical pharmacology scene has largely ditched cardiovascular medicine, its meetings now sporting huge sections devoted to neurological pharmacology and papers with such titles as *Adenosine A1245xxg receptors in the mouse hypothalamus are not up-regulated by 22 weeks of PVM55544 as much as adenosine A1245xxf receptors in the rat corpus striatum ... are ...* – and that *has* to be a good thing.

So the neurologist's position at our cocktail party may be changing. The thin, soft-spoken bespectacled guy in the corner whom nobody wants to talk to (not because he looks boring, you understand, but because his unsettling demeanour suggests that he analyses everything you say – looking boring is a coincidence) may well be feeling his way out of the shadows. He'll still drive an ageing slightly too big car of moderate pedigree, and will happily recount to any who'll listen its various faults and idiosyncrasies ... none of which he'll have bothered trying to fix.

So whether anyone as yet will want to talk to him ...

History and examination

There is a doctrine – well regarded in cognoscenti circles – that examination of a patient tells you *where* the problem is, while taking the history tells you the pathogenesis behind the problem. When it comes to neurology, this view is spot on. Take, for example, a stroke. Examination of the patient's limbs, speech and cranial nerves will tell you (if you know about these things) where the lesion is. In the hands of an expert, this can be mind-bogglingly precise. For example, a right hemiplegia plus a left facial (cranial nerve VII) palsy and a complete left lateral gaze palsy is *Foville's syndrome*, where the *nucleus* of the abducens (cranial nerve VI) in the dorsum of the pons is involved. If the lateral gaze problem is 'partial' (weakness rather than palsy), the lesion involves the *fascicle* rather than the nucleus and therefore is in the *ventral* part of the pons (a totally different syndrome – *Millard–Gubler*!). However, this tells you nothing about whether it was a bleed, a thrombosis, a tumour – or indeed traumatic. This we get from taking a history – in this scenario, almost entirely from speed of onset.

History

Headache
Headache shouldn't really be down as a neurological symptom. The cause is almost never neurological – but we don't have a 'stress and strainology' section, so this one is as good as any.

Arguably, headache is unique, being the only symptom which a patient will happily accept as not having a worrying organic origin (primary headache). Any other symptoms for which the doctor can find no explanation prompt the accusation 'So what's causing all the pains, then? Are you saying I'm making it all up?', but headaches without a cause seem to be acceptable. Indeed, I'll often use headache as an example for patients with joint/muscle pains for which I've found no 'organic' cause. *'Lots of people have headaches − but they don't have brain tumours or anything else actually going wrong in their head. But that doesn't mean anybody's saying they don't really have headaches and are making it all up. Joint and muscle pains can be the same.'*

Sometimes it helps. Other times, people insist that stress and strain can only cause pain in the head − not in the muscles, even though they'll admit it's easier to hold a muscle tense than to hold a brain tense. Pointing out that tension headaches may be caused by tension in the neck muscles is unlikely to get you anywhere. Brain strained, brain pained.

So what constitutes a worrying headache? Well, for a start, not one that's been the same for the past 25 years. Don't scoff. The 'new patients' at a general medical clinic are almost entirely made up of dizzy spells and variants on the headache theme.[2] The latter will include patients with a history of headaches for very many years − some with constant headache all day every day unchanged during all that time. If asked why they are presenting now, many will reveal that they've seen numerous physicians over the years with exactly the same symptoms.

Headaches in someone who doesn't get headaches are much more likely to be significant.

The nature and site of headaches may help. The 'tight band round the head' and the pain at the point of the vertex are both unlikely to be of sinister origin. Long-standing pain in the back of the neck going up into the occiput is most likely from cervical spine/muscles.

Most people with headache, of course, present because they believe they may have a brain tumour − and this is an entirely rational fear, despite not being mathematically likely.[3] The headache of tumour is basically the headache of increased intracranial pressure (from a 'space-occupying lesion' − SOL). Pain over the last two or three months ... gradual onset ... can't remember when it first started. Take them back to that time. Was it worse in the morning? SOL headaches often start as one which completely disappears shortly after getting up, only to return the next morning. Gradually worse. Gradually longer.

Accompanying nausea is a serious sign. Vomiting is later, and major − although this and the classic accompaniment of 'visual symptoms' also occur with migraines. Since part of the plan here is to separate out the stress/strain headaches from those with an 'organic' basis, to some extent the SOL and migraine do go together − and we come to:

---

[2] Most other symptoms are sent to the appropriate specialist. Headache isn't really neurological (I think I mentioned), and in any case neurologists usually brand themselves as 'tertiary referral' types − i.e. cases have to go through a hospital general physician before they'll even consider seeing them. So headaches go to the general medical clinic.

[3] Like flying in an aeroplane. The chances of crashing are remote (though 14 times as likely as winning the jackpot in the lottery!), but anyone who *doesn't* worry that 5000 tons of metal which only stays up in the sky by going too fast to fall down ... *might* not make it ... is clearly deranged.

> **Paradoxical Tip No. 1** If paracetamol clears your headache, it's *more* likely to have an organic basis.

The headache of a brain tumour in its early days will be obliterated by paracetamol, which will also help migraine. Stress headache, on the other hand, will often be entirely refractory even to strong analgesics.

The site of the pain is not always a major help, but will often be constant in the history, rather than flitting about, since it does depend on the site of the lesion to some extent.

Migraine[4] headaches are bizarre. It never ceases to amaze me how GPs can take a history of severe headaches plus vomiting plus scary visual episodes and confidently put it down to migraine when I'd have got out my CT scanner before you could say 'unnecessary X-ray exposure'. But such they do. And right they usually are. Experience, I guess – and one reason why any headache which *has* been sent up by such a GP needs to be taken seriously. I admit it does seem fairly easy once the patient's had a few episodes, but how can they diagnose it after the first one? The one-sided headache (he*mi-graine*) is obviously a clue, except that nobody ever has the one-sided headache. And I suppose the prodrome is a dead giveaway, if only anybody ever had the prodrome.

Temporal arteritis

We have to mention this. It's getting more common, but it's still rare, despite becoming a very trendy misdiagnosis. As with polymyalgia rheumatica, if a patient is less than 55 years old, think twice; if they are less than 50, think more than twice; if they are less than 45, simply dismiss it as a possibility.[5]

The headache is usually in the area of one of the temporal arteries (honest!). Severe. The patient has often been generally unwell (as in out of sorts rather than 'ill'), maybe even with fevers, off their food, grumpy, depressed[6] ... just not themselves. Often with aches and pains (and morning stiffness) elsewhere. Temporal arteritis is not the cause of a sudden headache in an otherwise well 60-year-old – and while it *can* occur with a normal ESR (check other markers such as CRP and immunoglobulins), it doesn't tend to. So, when none of the other features are actually present ... the headache is in the wrong place, the arteries aren't tender but are pulsatile,[7] and the ESR is minus 3 ... *why has the world suddenly decided that this has to be temporal arteritis until proven otherwise?*

The only explanation would appear to be that by doing so we can make headache the province of the rheumatologist. Note that while my medical paranoia

---

[4] Sorry, can't help with pronunciation. It's constantly changing whether 'my-grain' or 'mee-grain' will get you the job.

[5] Can't really say that. Never say 'never' in medicine. But we've got to stop people giving 60 mg prednisolone to 30-year-old women with headaches because *polymyalgia* sounds a bit like *fibromyalgia*.

[6] Careful when asking about the depression. Mention first that the diagnosis you're considering can make you feel depressed – otherwise the patient may take umbrage that 'you think this is all depression?'.

[7] I iterate – it is a common misconception that temporal arteritis makes the arteries pulsatile. In fact, it can make them palpable, and they may lose the pulsatility *that they normally have*. (It is a common misconception that *reiterate* means to *say again*; it actually means *to repeat again*.)

sees surgeons everywhere palming off all their problems on the physicians, my rheumatological paranoia sees physicians palming off their problems on rheumatologists. Much as the politically incorrect 'Irishman' (i.e. silly rustic) jokes are told in Ireland about 'Kerrymen', in Kerry about the punters from some small local village ... and so on ... until eventually one hyper-intelligent Mick at Number 42 gets a world of gags heaped upon him by everyone in his street – and I personally get to look after all the tough cases on the planet.

Sudden headache

The hit-on-the-back-of-the-head-by-a-baseball-bat[8] headache is classic for subarachnoid haemorrhage (SAH). Even below this intensity, sudden unexplained headache needs to be taken seriously. Statistics will tell you that SAH is always unlikely – even in the classic scenarios such as postcoital headache, where a recent study showed that only 10–20% of them will be caused by SAH ('*only*'!). The reason for the sudden blinding headache in the other 80% was not delineated.[9]

In my experience, features pointing to SAH – other than the suddenness of the headache – are difficult to define. SAH sufferers, however, may exhibit an indifference, almost surliness[10] – as if they can't be bothered with all these questions – so a vagueness in history here can be a positive pointer rather than a negative one.

Weakness/dizziness

More general medical fodder. Genuine weakness has to be distinguished from a fatigue–lethargy type of problem. And, indeed, pain. Site may help. 'Weakness all over' is unlikely to be neurological (and, I suppose, weakness down the left-hand side is unlikely to be lethargy), as is sudden weakness in the legs which recovers shortly afterwards. Weakness is one of the complaints that a patient with a very ... non-specific illness may complain of. It's worth going into such complaints in some detail. A blithe recording of 'weakness in the legs' or 'left arm weakness' in the case notes gives no real information to the next practitioner, or may push them down an entirely incorrect road. Taking a careful history can reveal pointers to specific diagnoses (e.g. slurring of speech or visual symptoms alongside hemiparesis).

Cynical Tip No. 12 Keep an ear open for 'creative' episodes that defy organic explanation (e.g. recurrent falls due to sudden painless loss of power with no alteration of consciousness and full recovery with magical avoidance of any injury at any time).

---

[8] Oddly, this is the UK description as well as the US one. Perhaps the image of whirling a cricket bat around someone's head seems so ... unwieldy.

[9] I believe the use of nitrates and related drugs as 'performance enhancers' was considered. Headache due to vasodilatation from nitrates has long been recognised – from the days when workers in explosives factories (TNT resembles GTN) developed headaches which settled as the week wore on (tachyphylaxis – the drug having less effect as the body gets used to it), only to reappear on the Monday morning after a weekend free of nitrate exposure; a concept now utilised as the 'nitrate-free period' in the treatment of angina, where patients may, for example, take off their nitrate patches overnight. An imaginative marketing of nitrate sprays as a benign alternative to mace in M'Lady's handbag (one squirt in the assailant's face – and *he* gets a headache) never caught on.

Histories of dizziness also have to be taken carefully. 'Dizzy' means different things to different people. Recently I saw a woman in her seventies with this complaint. Going into the story, what she was calling 'dizzy' was an increasing inability to concentrate/remember, and she was actually describing the signs of early dementia as 'dizziness'. Certainly it's worth starting by distinguishing the vertigo[11] (world spins round you, with or without nausea, with or without vomiting) of cerebellar or middle ear disease from the less specific 'light-headedness' of everything else under the sun (neurological, respiratory, cardiac, spurious ...)

Next – when does it happen? When you stand up (maybe postural hypotension)? When you turn your head (maybe cervical spondylosis[12])? When you're having sex (maybe just fortuitous choice of partner)? Accompanied/preceded by chest pain ... palpitations ... coughing ... food ... fasting ... It can be anything. Dizziness has to be taken along with the rest of the story before you have any idea what's behind it.

Blackouts and seizures

The first thing to determine is whether there was indeed loss of consciousness (LOC). Patients' ideas of blackouts vary from a four-day spell they can remember nothing about (including where they hid the loot) to a millisecond's loss of concentration while following the plot of *EastEnders*.

An actual LOC is always significant, though many benign causes exist. A story of what the patient was doing in the short and medium term before is *hugely* helpful – whether this be obvious, like injecting heroin, putting out a forest fire, seeing who could hold their breath under the water for longest ... or more subtle, like finishing exercise, turning their head sharply, having a coughing fit (cough syncope), going to the loo to empty their bladder – especially during the night (micturition syncope), standing in a very warm room ... or even negatives like not having their lunch, not taking their steroid tablets, or not avoiding a lamp-post. As with chest pain, patients will always start off by telling you that they were 'doing nothing'. Persuade them to humour you.

Take the story first of everything that *the patient* felt – not what he or she was told by others, or their interpretation of what he or she had. Only then should you get some history from witnesses – whether or not this be via the patient themselves.[13] Don't get too optimistic, though. It's amazing how useless witnesses tend to be. No one ever takes a pulse during the episode, no one ever tells the patient how long he was out, or notices what colour the patient went.

Patients may feel hot or sweaty before blackouts (vaso-vagal), feel hungry, have pains in the chest, palpitations ... (all a bit like dizziness) or may have an 'aura', which might suggest a seizure. Take them gently through the story – were they

---

[10] I have tried referring to this insight as 'Larkin's sign', but colleagues and students unanimously assumed that this referred to a comparison with my demeanour, rather than my having discovered the sign.

[11] No more equal to a fear of heights than 'diarrhoea' is equal to a fear of flying.

[12] Hence all patients with dizziness should be referred to the rheumatologist.

[13] OK then, politically correct word users who don't want me to use 'himself' ... should this be 'themselves' or, oddly, 'themself'?

standing or sitting, doing something or watching TV?[14] If they did lose consciousness, where did they wake up?

Cynical Tip No. 13   It's a good idea to go through this completely before
picking up on any discrepancies. Where the patient woke up can be particularly inexplicable. Patients may describe the ambulancemen coming in
and stretching them out, taking them in the ambulance to the hospital, where
they then woke up …

If they were confused when they woke up, how long did this take to settle?
Afterwards, did they have any headache or generalised muscle pain (seizure)?
It's also usual to ask about tongue (or lip) biting or urinary incontinence when
attempting to diagnose generalised seizures – though these findings are neither
ubiquitous in seizures nor exclusive to them (e.g. urinary incontinence can occur
in vaso-vagal attacks … mind you, is such a vaso-vagal a seizure?). Once the
confusion went away, did they feel absolutely normal, or perhaps tired or washed-
out? The absence of confusion or tiredness is a greater pointer against generalised
seizures than the absence of tongue biting or incontinence.

When patients present with a recurring symptom, be it seizures or angina, they
often respond to questions about the current event in general terms.

'How long did it last?'
'Oh, they usually go on for about 20 minutes.'

Get them to focus on one clear episode. With seizures I usually get them to tell me
about the first one they ever had, and also all about the most recent episode.

A quick résumé of seizures may help here.

Part of the definition of epilepsy is 'recurrent seizures' – so one seizure does
not epilepsy make. Seizures themselves are usually classified into partial and
generalised. The latter include the classic *'grand mal'* seizures – now described
as 'generalised tonic–clonic seizures' (GTCS) – where the subject goes through
the phases of all the muscles going rigid ('tonic' – surprisingly, the bit when the
tongue gets bitten), followed by the general shaking of arms/legs ('clonic'). This is
always accompanied by loss of awareness (essentially LOC – even if the patient
is moving). If the patient can remember all of that shaking stuff then it wasn't a
seizure (one organic option being a rigor). The LOC usually goes on for some time
after the shaking has stopped. The patient awakes confused – perhaps for a further
10–30 minutes – and then may have tiredness/headache as described above.

Partial seizures depend on which part of the brain is involved. An occipital
seizure might consist solely of visual symptoms such as flashing lights, an
olfactory lobe seizure might consist of an odd smell, and a parietal seizure might
involve an episode of disorientation. More often some adjacent structures will be

---

[14] There is a subgroup of epileptic subjects – the same ones that are prone to seizures at strobe-lit
discos, if such things still exist – whose seizures are precipitated by watching a TV change channels
while they move towards it! Having something to do with the connections across the brain via the
corpus callosum, these can sometimes be avoided by closing one eye when either approaching
the TV or changing channels. The trick is to persuade the patient to believe a word of this. (I believe
they can also be helped by slicing through the corpus callosum – my way just seems easier.)

'enrolled', and other symptoms including abnormal movements may occur. If the subject remains aware of this, it's a *simple* partial seizure, but if the episode progresses to loss of awareness, this is a *complex* partial seizure. In many patients with such problems, some or most of their seizures will progress to full-blown GTCS – when they will be known as secondary generalised seizures. The classic example of these is the 'Jacksonian seizure',[15] where the shaking begins in – for example – one finger, spreads to the whole arm and then to the rest of the body.

Defining the type of seizure is important when it comes to anticonvulsant therapy (among other paradoxes, partial seizures are more difficult to eradicate) – so taking a precise history is important, particularly in a GTCS when you wish to determine whether it is primary or secondary. The beginning of the attack carries the main clues. An aura suggests a secondary GTCS – the nature of the aura depending on the focus of the partial seizure (which may or may not have some recognisable lesion as its basis). The aura is essentially the same as a small seizure which doesn't spread, and may consist of flashing lights, an odd smell, an odd feeling in the stomach, or a déjà-vu phenomenon (usually associated with temporal lobe epilepsy – TLE was possibly the first recognised of all partial seizures and the one most generally known about, leading to its erroneously being considered by many as synonymous with partial epilepsy). Patients may thus describe, with some surprise, episodes where they had the aura but then 'nothing happened'. Another feature that suggests partial seizures is 'automatisms' – apparently purposeful movements such as switching on a light, removing a sweater (usually one's own) or brushing an imaginary spider off the lap, of which the patient is unaware and which they don't remember afterwards.

This clinical differentiation is borne out by electroencephalographic (EEG) studies in which generalised seizures are seen to start 'all over' the brain, whereas the partial seizures start at a focus and then gradually spread out to other areas. The extent of the spread is reflected in the clinical extent of the seizure.

EEGs also help to dispel some of the myths surrounding 'petit mal' seizures – everybody's favourite.[16] These very simple episodes consisting of a few seconds' loss of awareness with instantaneous recovery (and that's it!) are primary *generalised* seizures – *not* partial. They almost never occur in adults. Occasionally they persist from childhood, but more frequently the problem either dies out or converts into another form of seizure. Most adults who say that they suffer from *'petit mal'* either have partial seizures, perhaps diagnosable from a history of aura such as a déjà-vu phenomenon (usually associated with temporal lobe epilepsy – TLE was possibly the first recognised of all partial seizures and the one most generally known about, leading to its erroneously being considered by many as synonymous with partial epilepsy) – or do not have epilepsy at all.

Myoclonic seizures ('myoclonic jerks'[17]) are sudden movements of one or two muscles, most frequently in the morning (so persistently dropping your breakfast coffee is almost pathognomonic). They are worth looking out for as they may accompany other forms of epilepsy, and can be exacerbated by some therapies, such as carbamazepine.

---

[15] Named after (John) Hughlings Jackson, 1835–1911 – the 'father' of modern epilepsy thinking.
[16] Surely a testimony to the appealing Gallic ring of *'petit mal'*. Since the approved term is now 'absence seizure', this interpretation is supported by the inexplicable insistence of many on pronouncing this 'absongsssss' *à la français*.
[17] Not to be confused with any abusive term for our friends the neurosurgeons.

A careful history of the episodes themselves is thus the most important thing, though we usually include some background information. Although most epilepsy is probably due to some indefinable perinatal damage we don't yet understand, there may be stories of 'difficult birth' (formerly 'blue baby' or 'cord wrapped round neck') or being hit by a swing as a child (though such injuries, if short of causing a fracture, are unlikely ever to cause seizures). More important than these episodes is probably some underlying propensity to seizures. At least part of this is genetic. Asked if they have any family history of epilepsy, a patient may reply 'Not really. My father had seizures, but he had his skull fractured in an accident at work.' In fact this patient *is* more likely to develop a seizure disorder than someone with no such family history. Following a skull fracture (or stroke, or major alcohol abuse) most people do not develop seizures. Those who do have some pre-disposition and this, to some extent, will be reflected in their family.

Pseudoseizures

It took some time before we were allowed to talk about pseudoseizures out loud. Only once we emphasised that patients weren't 'pretending to have a seizure' (although lots of others do) did the politically correct establishment[18] let the epilepsy-treating world discuss this phenomenon. Usually (but not always) pseudo-seizures occur in people who suffer from a seizure disorder — that is, they also suffer from true seizure events. In a pseudoseizure the patient may have all of the features of a true seizure ... tonic–clonic phases with shaking ... apparent loss of awareness ... etc. However, EEG telemetry (simultaneous video recording of the patient with EEG recording of 'brainwaves') will demonstrate that these episodes are not initiated by any 'electrical' event in the brain. In most cases the subject isn't 'pretending to have a seizure', as they do appear to lose control of the episode. Many patients will voluntarily discuss their two different types of seizure. One which comes out of the blue, at any time, and others which tend to be brought on by stress and/or anger and which they find themselves drifting into — sometimes being able to abort these by strength of will if they catch themselves early enough. Particularly in those without other seizure disorder, an association has been suggested between pseudoseizures and past sexual abuse (some of the 'seizure' movements may be indicative). For those who do have a seizure disorder, my own belief is that as children, when under conditions of stress/family disharmony, they 'learned' that having a seizure would make the world right ... everybody would love them again ... and this becomes an ingrained behaviour pattern as the years go on — which they don't actually control.

Cynical Tip No. 14 If a patient is having a pseudoseizure (or indeed a feigned seizure — not the same thing) then they will usually resist any attempt to open their eyes. The eyes of patients who are having genuine seizures, on the other hand, can usually be easily opened by the examiner.

---

[18] Medicine had its political correctness before it ever became trendy. This concerned only the discussion of patients, where no one was allowed to suggest aloud in public that patients might ever, possibly ever, be 'putting it on' — even though it was a universally acknowledged truth in private. As with most current forms of PC, it was all based on appearances — the fact that no one can accuse you of bias, prejudice, etc. being more important than whether you actually have any ...

Anaesthesia/paraesthesia

Patients will say it feels 'numb'. First find out whether this is indeed the medical idea of numbness (i.e. anaesthesia – it almost never is) or some pins-and-needles variant. Find out exactly where it is, when it occurs and how long it lasts. 'Trapped nerve' is a favourite diagnosis of patients.[19] If that is their preferred diagnosis, the 'numbness' will be painful. A precise history of the site will help you to decide if a nerve distribution is indeed involved. Patients with dubious stories of paraesthesia will almost always have these in fictitious nerve distributions which end at joints. Unfortunately, so do a lot of non-fictitious distributions. Further detailing may, however, produce some inconsistencies.

Cynical Tip No. 15   Ask whether a paraesthesia goes all around a section of limb (e.g. forearm). I can't define myself what that would mean, but dubious patients spot a trap and hedge their bets unconvincingly.

Cynical Tip No. 16   Patients don't know the 'anatomical position' – you know, the one with your hands by your side, palms facing forward. In this position, root distributions make sense, but laymen think of the arm with palms down, so created paraesthesiae will often 'jump' (e.g. from C5 to C8).

Carpal tunnel syndrome (a genuine nerve entrapment – median N at the wrist) is usually worse at night – with pain as well as paraesthesia. Relief is sometimes obtained by hanging the arm down from the bed. Less specific ... all over ... variable paraesthesia is more likely to be part of a 'pain syndrome' such as fibromyalgia.

Again, learn the distributions from a proper book. The following observations only make sense in conjunction with one.

Roots

C7	Middle finger. The rest of the arm C5–T2 just falls into place around it.
Thoracics	Back higher than front.
T6	Nipple.
T10	Navel (don't let pendulous breasts fool you there's still a T7–9).
L2–5	Out-in–in-out.

Nerves

Median	Thumb $+ 2\frac{1}{2}$ fingers.
Common peroneal	Foot drop. Get the patient to attempt everting the foot as well as attempting dorsiflexion. Partial palsies may be picked up.

---

[19] And of osteopaths/chiropractors. Second only to 'malalignment of the spine', which is present in 105% of people attending an osteopath.

> **Cynical Tip No. 17**   Hemianaesthesia involving the face must surely be more commonly psychogenic than anything else (certainly in the absence of other signs).

Neurological examination

Cranial nerves
Absolutely spanking fun to examine. Only time for a few tips.

I   Olfactory
Don't use smelling salts (ammonia) or other irritant. These are recognisable by their irritation of the nasal mucosa (trigeminal nerve [V]).

II   Optic
Acuity. As long as they can read (and can therefore do the tests), anything more precise is not your problem. Remember that they've got two eyes (unless, of course, they haven't, in which case make sure that you notice).

Colour. A harmless drudge – unless you're an airline pilot or ship's master.[20]

Visual fields. You're allowed to sit on the bed! 'Confrontation' means comparing the patient's visual field of, for example, their right eye with your left while facing them. This actually is only true of the nasal field as the temporal field goes back more than $100°$ [21] – so unless your arm is 11% longer than infinity (according to Stephen Hawking, almost seven feet), you'll have to include a bringing-the-wiggling-finger-from-behind-the-patient's-back manoeuvre into your repertoire to pick up minimal reductions of lateral fields (though causes of such escape me at the moment).

The wiggling finger itself is worthy of comment, since getting the patient to correctly indicate when it stops confirms that they are indeed seeing it. Reasons for a patient's being deceitful may fail to spring to mind (perhaps fighter pilots trying to hold on to their jobs in obsolete pre-radar aircraft or bouncers or bodyguards or … oooh! – air … traffic … control …), but some patients, including one in yesterday's membership exam, with for example, dementia may be vague, tired or just trying to please.

Visual fields are worth taking time over. The cursory examination where the patient gives a perfunctory 'now' at some random point as a wobbly finger is swept across their eyeline is no help to anyone. OK, there's rarely an abnormality, but there's no point in just going through the motions of doing a test.

Know the causes of the standard visual field losses. Dead simple. If you can draw the diagram: … coming right up.

---

[20] It always seemed odd that the two colours most commonly confused by 'colour-blind' subjects are chosen to represent port and starboard sides of sailing and aircraft … presumably the person who decided this would be only too happy to have the occasional traffic light turned upside-down.
[21] This surprises lots of people – but just try it. All to do with the eyeball being … a ball.

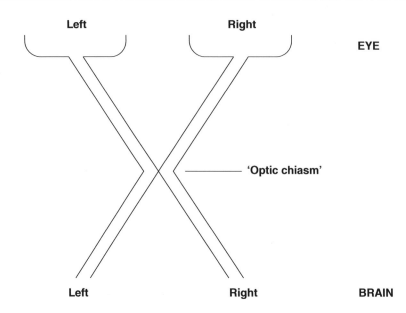

And remember that the right half of each fundus sees the left half of the world: You'll be fine ... but I'll mention two things.

1 Bitemporal hemianopia ... loss of both temporal fields (duh!) ... associated with pituitary tumours or aneurysm in the area of chiasm ... *isn't* 'tunnel vision'.
2 Patients with homonomous hemianopia are not so highly trained as yourself (even), and do not realise that this is the problem. They will always think that they have lost the sight of the eye on that side.

Scotoma(ta)

These are difficult to find unless you really spend some time − or use that big fancy machine thing.[22] The classic (which I have yet to see) is the extension of the 'physiological blind spot',[23] being the earliest scotoma in glaucoma.

At this point it is necessary to leave the quasi-systematic approach to the cranial nerves in order to have a quick squint at pupils.

Pupils
Both big

OK, there's all the standard causes − drugs, such as amphetamines, anti-cholinergics (including tricyclics, antihistamines, phenothiazines), alcohol, cannabis, local drugs (eyedrops such as atropine/homatropine, tropicamide[24]). Also major

---

[22] Bjerrum's screen. It has only just occurred to me that all testing of the optic nerve involves rarely used eponyms − Bjerrum, Ishihara, Snellen ... Wiggly ...

[23] To emphasise the difficulty, it's worth reminding ourselves of the existence of this with the childhood exercise of drawing a black spot on a big piece of paper, with a cross drawn about 10 cm to the right of it. Focusing on the spot with your right eye (shut the other one!), hold the paper at arm's length and move it slowly towards you. At some point the cross will disappear − as you're trying to see it with your optic disc. Keep going and it reappears. You go through life oblivious to this, and patients can have quite large scotomata without realising (you could say they have a bl- ... but we won't).

[24] The commonest reason for large pupils in an exam is that the organiser has put drops in them.

brain problems including death (few medical phrases have the solemn permanence of 'fixed and dilated'). But with a bit of imagination you can come up with:

- pleasure – 'Is that a midriatic you've got in your socket, or are you just pleased to see me?'
- darkness – scary in infra-red footage
- dark eyes – it is now proven that dark eyes have larger pupils than blue ones. This – along with the 'BellaDonna' sobriquet for atropine used by ladies of the Court to make their pupils larger and therefore make them appear more beautiful – has been viewed by many (well, the wife) as incontrovertible proof that brunettes are more attractive than blondes.

Both small
- Particularly bright room.
- Particularly ugly blonde.

Oh, all right:

- pontine haemorrhage
- opiate ingestion (including lesser ones such as dihydrocodeine and dextropropoxyphene[25])
- pilocarpine eyedrops (glaucoma).

One big, one small
First decide which one's abnormal by checking the reaction to light[26] – the one which doesn't react is almost always the culprit.

Big one is abnormal	*Well* subject	IIIrd nerve palsy (often partial)
	Ill subject	Major brain lesion including raised ICP from *anything* ('false localising sign')
	Exam subject	Mydriatic in eye. In fact, since this is usually dilated so that you can see diabetic retinopathy, then the smartest[27] answer for the cause of a large pupil in an exam is ... diabetes!

---

[25] Dextropropoxyphene. Until recently, a great drug to know about. The opiate in co-proxamol (the old 'Distalgesic'). Easy to swallow, and easy to remember the constituents – paracetamol 325 mg, dextropropoxyphene 32.5 mg – yet you will astound your peers and masters with this knowledge. Also an enzyme inhibitor which increases the actions of other drugs by inhibiting their breakdown – it can play havoc with the effects of warfarin, theophylline, anticonvulsants or contraceptives (oral – the half-life of condoms is unaltered), particularly since being an analgesic it is taken sporadically. These complications plus a tendency to cause cardiac problems in overdose have just this very minute caused its sudden withdrawal from the market. Almost a shame, really. Particularly since it's a much better analgesic than it's given credit for.

[26] Remember to shine the light from the side (and twice for consensual). Patients genuinely focus on a small light in front of them, producing constriction of the pupil due to the accommodation reflex – thus masking an Argyll–Robertson pupil (accommodating, but doesn't react – the Med School mnemonic regarding its provenance needs no mention here). I have witnessed this – in the enviable position of registrar-organiser of the MRCP, having to explain to an *examiner* why his technique wasn't eliciting the desired effect. Nice feeling ... being a registrar for ten years ...

[27] Actually the 'most likely correct' answer – not necessarily smart.

Small one is abnormal	Horner's syndrome (sympathetic chain damage from high thoracic lesion such as tumour or aneurysm … 'reduced everything', i.e. reduced size of pupil, reduced size of eye (?!) reduced amount of sweat that side … blah de blah … almost always partial …) Pilocarpine drops in eye (glaucoma therapy).

Consensual light reflex – I'll deal with this in the next edition.

III, IV, VI   Oculomotor, trochlear, abducens

These are always considered together, though their actions go beyond the intrinsic muscles of the eye.

Eye movements shouldn't simply be tested along the midlines. One suggested alternative is to include diagonal movements – which I am happy to dismiss since any time I ask a candidate to explain their significance I am met by a flummoxed, silent stare. That leaves us with the 'figure of H' approach – like the gear lever on a car. You get the patient to look to the left, then move the eyes up and down, followed by looking to the right and then up and down.[28] When the eye is abducted (looking out sideways) the superior rectus and the inferior rectus move the pupil up and down, respectively. When the pupil is adducted (looks at your nose), the oblique muscles predominantly perform these functions – and since they're inserted oddly, the eye is moved up by the *inferior* oblique and down by the *superior*. Thus the 'figure of H' manoeuvre can pinpoint single muscle abnormalities. All you have to remember is that the lateral rectus is supplied by VI, the superior oblique by IV, and all the rest by III – and you're laughing. There are numerous mnemonics for this – the simple 'L_6SO_4' being favoured by my own chemistry-orientated Med School.[29]

As the patient follows your finger, always remember to ask if they see double at any point – which may help you to spot minor weaknesses. Sixth nerve palsies give diplopia looking laterally in that direction, while a fourth nerve palsy may give diplopia looking down (I diagnosed an isolated fourth nerve palsy in a close relative over the phone when she told me she'd tripped down the back stairs (two steps) twice in three days for no reason).

> **Cynical Tip No. 18**   If the patient complains of diplopia, try them with one eye closed. While rare causes of diplopia with one eye do exist (severe astigmatism or … er …), it is most likely that anyone with diplopia in one eye is making it up.

---

[28] Sometimes (rarely) they can only do this while following a finger, sometimes only when not (i.e. 'look to the left' – all too sophisticated for this book … concerning internuclear connections … cortical control … all that sort of interesting stuff).

[29] Making up one's own mnemonics is most profitable. It also adds further zest to a 'game' I devised with colleagues trained at other Med Schools. You give them your mnemonic (the more obtuse the better) and '20 questions' to work out what it's for (yes … it does suddenly seem a bit saddo, but it's so difficult to see train numbers these days). Among other things, you can compare levels of racism and licentiousness in the faculties. While these qualities are deliberately introduced to increase memorability, facial nerve branches might have been just as memorable if a zebra, not a Zulu, had done the deed. My own favourite rheumatological mnemonic is *SEW*, which I invented to help me memorise the order of the joints in the upper limb …

V   Trigeminal

There are three branches – *ophthalmic, maxillary* and *mandibular* (mnemonic: 'OMM' …) – and three modalities to check.

- *Sensory*. Lightly touch each of the three areas on each side and ensure that the patient feels these normally.
- *Motor*. Feel masseters clenching teeth (just below and in front of the tragus). Get the patient to open their mouth against resistance (your fist placed under their chin[30]). One of the three big '50–50' questions in cranial nerve examination – if one side is weak, which way will the chin go?
- *Smart-ass*. Corneal reflex. This is mediated by a long looping 'tail' of the Vth nucleus, so can be surprisingly involved in lesions 'lower down' in the brain (e.g. those damaging IX–X–XI). It is a very sensitive test. The brain's plan is … touch my cornea, I'll immediately blink to protect it. (Indeed, if you've ever had the optician try to measure your ocular pressures with that air-puff thing and she has to try 40 times, it becomes clear that the brain blinks *before* anything (even air) touches it. Obvious best plan really – but very clever.) Our plan is to check the integrity of this reflex by wisping up a small amount of cotton wool and **gently** touching **once** the very edge of the cornea. The patient should blink (doubly smart consensual move – as opposed to winking – for which we don't give the nervous system enough credit). There is **no** need to stroke the cotton repeatedly – or once over the cornea. If the patient doesn't blink – that's odd. You *might* just try it once again to confirm.

A corneal reflex – while not at the embarrassment level of a rectal examination – is probably at the invasive level where in an exam one would suggest its necessity in the first instance, and carry on only if required. Oddly, the alternative method of blowing lightly across the open eye is arguably less invasive, but carries an 'ick' factor which makes us avoid it.

VII   Facial

Check for wrinkling the brows, shutting the eyes tight (you shouldn't be able to overcome this legally), smiling or pulling up the corners of mouth.[31] In an exam, no one will ask you to examine the facial nerves without demanding your method of distinguishing an upper motor neuron (UMN) lesion from a lower one (LMN). Only two things to remember. One is the simple drawing overleaf.[32]

As we can see, the right cortex pretty much supplies the entire left facial nucleus so the left side of the face is controlled by the right side of the brain. However, it does drop off a small supply to the upper part of the 'ipsilateral' right facial nucleus. Similarly, the left facial nucleus does get *some* innervation to its *upper* part from its ipsilateral left cortex. So, while a disruption at 'A' (LMN lesion) will

---

[30] As with sitting on the bed during visual fields, I believe that this is the only time you are allowed to do this.

[31] As with finger following, there are some subtleties here. Depending on which part of the cortex is impaired, patients may be unable to smile when asked, but can respond to a joke with a wide grin. The opposite may also occur – supposedly rare – but in my experience present in more than 75% of the normal population.

[32] OK. Schematic and ultimately inaccurate – but still worth an International Award. (Is Russell Square really south-west of Farrington, or Victoria due west of the Embankment?)

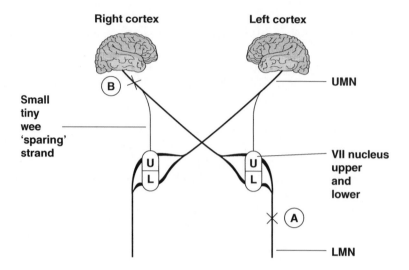

totally obliterate the left facial nerve function, a disruption around 'B' (UMN lesion) will thoroughly reduce the left nerve function, but some function of the upper nucleus will be 'spared'.

And this is the second thing to know. The meaning of 'sparing'. The often-described 'sparing' of the upper face muscles in a UMN lesion does not mean that they are normal. This is the 'sparing' championed by the bad guy in *Batman* or *Zorro* or *DieHard 42* – where he spares your life, but cuts off your leg, throws you in a cage and runs off with your wife and/or daughter. The eyes and forehead will *not* work normally in most UMN lesions (e.g. you will be able to open their eyes despite their best efforts – whereas with a complete LMN the patient will not be able to close their eyes in the first place[33]) – so don't find a degree of weakness here and erroneously decide that the lesion is LMN.

VIII   Auditory/vestibular ... vestibulocochlear

Basic hearing ability in each ear can be tested by whispering (so difficult to find a ticking watch nowadays) while the patient rubs the other tragus into the appropriate external meatus (tricky to explain to the patient in common parlance – can't think of an everyday word for the tragus for a start).

More precise testing needs the tuning fork. There are three variously available in medical wards (and occasionally in surgical wards, but only to stir the tea). All are 'C' and their frequencies are therefore powers of two[34] i.e. 128 Hz, 256 Hz and 512 Hz. The best for hearing tests is 512 Hz, the best for vibrational sense (qnv) is 128 Hz – so most wards make the compromise 256 Hz available (actually most wards have lost it, but this is the theory).

---

[33] The basis of Bell's phenomenon in Bell's palsy (VII LMN), where the patient's nervous system looks as if it's perpetually trying to tuck the eye up behind an eyelid which is unable to close.

[34] Which makes me wonder. Was the 'standard' musical key of C (no black notes on the piano!) decided by some ancient scientist/mathematician? Or does it just feel right to the human ear? To further complicate things, 'concert pitch' for orchestras is now defined around 'A' at 440 Hz. This in fact makes middle C about 261 Hz, not 256. But the 'Standard A' has been moved up twice over the years, from 435, first to 439, then to 440 in 1939. If it was back at 435, C would be around 256 – and in keeping with the 'scientific' scale. But it isn't. All very confusing. Is this why 'rap' just doesn't sound right?

Rinné's test

It initially surprises us to be told that we hear a tuning fork better when it's held to our ear than when the base is pressed against the mastoid – but give God (or whoever we attribute the ear's design to) *some* credit. So, normally, once the fading note has died at the mastoid, switching to the ear-hole will make it audible again (and not vice versa). Confusingly (though the alternative would be worse), normality (air conduction better than bone) is called 'Rinné negative'. *Per se*, it tells you little about hearing in the ear. However, in conjunction with knowing which ear hears poorly (the whispering), it helps to define the problem. If a 'deaf' ear has an abnormal Rinné's then the 'air conduction' mechanics of the ear must be impaired. If Rinné's is normal in a bad ear, then the auditory nerve should be the problem.

Weber's test is really just a bit of fun for confirmation. A tuning fork pressed against the forehead in the midline will normally be 'heard' as if it's ... in the midline. If there is nerve damage in the left ear, it will appear to be heard on the right. If there are air-conduction problems in the left ear, then the lack of extraneous noise from nurses and biscuit sellers in the left ear will make the central tuning fork buzz more prominent in the left ear – the 'bad' ear.

Cynical Tip No. 19   No tests are perfect – and conflicting evidence from Rinné's and Weber's tests may have no real significance (theoretically you should believe Rinné), but having found an apparent air conduction deafness on the left ... when one moves on to Weber's test, a dubious patient may intuitively say that he hears it better on the right.

The vestibular component of nerve VIII is dealt with in a perfunctory fashion under vertigo and nystagmus.

IX, X, XI   Glossopharyngeal, vagus, spinal accessory

These three have also been lumped together so much that their various functions have merged into a blur in the minds of most physicians (... well ... myself, anyway). This is understandable, since their actions do combine to perform the two functions of swallowing and speaking. Furthermore, the nuclei themselves are all in the one lump in the brain – such that problems in the area are usually put down to a 'bulbar palsy'[35] (though the area seems to be rarely referred to as 'the bulb') rather than individual nerves.

IX.   The glossopharyngeal nerve supplies sensation (including taste) to the posterior third of the tongue,[36] but its function – intertwined with the non-autonomic functions of the vagus (**X**) – is usually tested by noting the position of the uvula and its movement on getting the patient to say 'aaaaah!' (one of the few

---

[35] Or 'pseudobulbar palsy' when of UMN provenance. Distinguished by the accompanying emotional lability and 'hot-potato' or 'Donald-Duck' speech. Classic causes include motor neuron disease and multiple sclerosis, though surely most common are bilateral ischaemic 'strokes' – potentially very small in themselves – affecting this area. The problem presents itself at the time of the second stroke.

[36] The front two-thirds gets touch sensation from the trigeminal and taste from an extra branch of the facial (*chorda tympani*). Two pieces of information I've never actually used.

times you get to behave like the doctor in a TV series). The direction it moves in is the second big 50–50. (Only do 'gag reflex' if really necessary.)

XI.   Specific testing is of the sternomastoid – the *left* sternomastoid turning the head to the *right*. So this is tested vs. the pressure of your hand against the right side of the chin, your other hand feeling the left sternomastoid (to make sure it's doing the job – in its absence the pterygoids (CN V) can make a decent fist of the same movement) and ask the patient to turn their head to the right. (**Accidental Contrariness No. 2** – they will always begin by turning their head to the left.) Shoulder-shrugging is also XI, but less fun.

XII Hypoglossal.   Supplies the muscles of the tongue. The third and final big 50–50.

Cranial nerves – fallout

Nystagmus
Noooooooooooo! Far too tricky. All the clear-cut ones like rotating/ocillatory nystagmus (constant flickering of the eyes accustomed to using their peripheral vision[37]) and ataxic nystagmus (nothing to do with the cerebellum; on looking to the side, there's nystagmus in the abducting eye with some failure of adduction in the other. It's due to an intranuclear ophthalmoplegia – a problem in the medial longitudinal faciculus which joins III and VI in the side of the *adducting* eye – usually associated with multiple sclerosis) are rare.

We're left with all the cerebellum/middle ear/mid-brainstem causes which are really complicated. Which eye is worse?/looking which way?/going on for how long?/accompanied by what else? ... can only be added up by a proper doctor. I refuse to go and read a book so that I can pretend to know about it by writing down what the other guy says. Besides, how am I to know he's right? I might be perpetuating a false assumption. He might be making it up. At best he's probably copied it from some other guy who might be making it up ... or who copied it from someone else who's granny told him when he was a kid that when *she* was a kid she'd been told that spiky eye movements meant your cerebellum was damaged ... by someone who she thought might have been making it up ...

But I should mention nomenclature. Nystagmus 'to the right' refers to the fast phase (the jerk or saccade which recovers position from the previous drift) and not the direction in which the eye is looking. This usually comes to the same thing. Try it yourself. Look as far as you can to the right. It's a pain. Your eye starts to drift towards pleasant centralness and you have to jerk it back out. This is the basis of 'gaze-evoked nystagmus', a normal occurrence at $>45°$ in many people. Most forms of jerk nystagmus from drugs, brainstem, cerebellar lesions, etc., are an exaggeration of this.

Of further interest is the 'Hall–Pyke' manoeuvre and its variants in patients complaining of vertigo. Pushing their head back and then rotating to look down

---

[37] Classically those working in the dark such as coal miners. The cones of the central retina are more precise but less sensitive in the dark than the peripheral rods. Supposedly also occurred in fighter pilots of the Second World War who were trained to use their peripheral vision at night and flew with their eyes permanently moving from side to side. All things considered, not common nowadays.

may induce their vertigo symptoms plus observable nystagmus. This is most notably associated with 'benign positional vertigo' – thought to be due to debris in the semicircular canals[38] and it certainly suggests a vestibular reason above all others.

Nystagmus can be difficult to spot, never mind interpret. Very fine examples are occasionally spotted from movements of the optic disc when using ...

The ophthalmoscope

Patient examination
There is no obvious place to deal with this treacherous instrument, so we shall do so here. It is used in the examination of the pupils, though a pen-torch is much superior to its fragile light, and the only required advice vis-à-vis cranial nerves is to push the button to make the light come on. A few other tips:

1   Bring your own. It takes forever to get used to an ophthalmoscope.
2   Learn to breathe through your nose. Fundoscopy is a major cross-invasion of personal space, and you'll see many practitioners emerge as if they'd swum an underwater length of the Olympic Pool.
3   Start off with a +10/15 lens from a distance. That way you get to see the abnormalities in the front of the eye – including a crisp view of the cataract that will later obscure your view of the fundus.
4   'Move in', bringing the positivity down.
5   If you can't focus on the fundus, see if the patient has spectacles with a severe prescription and try to emulate this on the ophthalmoscope. If necessary, examine their glasses. Reading glasses have convex lenses (+) which magnify things. Myopic people have concave glasses (−) which make things smaller.[39] If this doesn't work, examine the patient through their own spectacles (though macula will be almost impossible owing to reflection).
6   Once you find a vessel, follow it to the optic disc to see if it's all swollen and mottled (papilloedema). If you think that the disc 'may be blurred', it's *probably* fine.[40]

Examination examination
In an exam, you're not looking for papilloedema unless the organiser has absolutely no sense of propriety. Exam patients for fundoscopy have diabetes or hypertension or both (unless they're chatting happily to the organising registrar, in which case they are a 'ringer' and their eye is normal). These are distinguishable from each other because the diabetic fundus has haemorrhages and exudates, while the hypertensive fundus has ... exudates and haemorrhages.

It's not easy.

---

[38] There is a suggested treatment where you scrunch the patient's head round the angles like a demon barber (would), designed to drain off the debris by manoeuvring it through the three perpendicular canals. Very entertaining to watch.
[39] My favourite scientific blunder in literature was always *Lord of the Flies*, where Piggy's glasses were used to make fire by concentrating the sun's rays. Since Piggy was short-sighted, the lens would *spread* the heat more soothingly across the paper. My big-screen equivalent is all those noisy battles in the vacuum of space.

But the examiner is going to pretend he can tell the difference (because it's down in his chitty), so you need a plan. One such plan would be to learn to tell one from the other – but that never worked for me. 'Hard exudates and haemorrhages – diabetes; soft exudates and flame haemorrhages – hypertension.' Pah! *They all look the same*. Or, more correctly, *they all look different*, which comes to the same thing. An alternative plan might be to spot the 'fundus patient' as you move round the exam area (they'll be the one with the ophthalmoscope beside them who's trying to read a newspaper propped up ten feet away against the window). Catch their eye. Smile at them. Keep doing this every chance you get. They'll start smiling back. By the time you're being asked to examine them, they'll be grinning at you like a long-lost nephew. The examiner will spot this and move you to an alternative patient.[41] Thus, instead of trying to decide via an alien contraption through a 3-mm space using a 1-mm light beam whether a yellow/red blob the size of a pinhead is hard or soft, you'll be taken to an RA/OA hand where you pretty much decide whether a blob the size of an entire eyeball is hard or soft. *And* you get to feel it.[42] If you still can't get it right, devil mend you. Particularly if, as you leave, you finally recognise the fundus patient as your long-neglected Auntie Jeannie, the one who you weren't supposed to bring chocolates because of her diabetes ...

Limbs
Oh ... sorry ... the big 50–50s.

V Opening mouth vs. resistance – chin goes towards the *bad* side (think as if muscles could *push*).

IX–X Say 'aaaah!' – the uvula moves towards the *good* side (think of the palate as your arms crossed over, hands clasped and hanging down like the uvula). Compare what happens when both arms pull up and only one arm pulls up.

XII 'Push out your tongue' – the tongue moves towards the *bad* side (again, think as if the muscles could push).

Limbs
Arms and legs may be examined for *tone, power, coordination* and *sensation*. Not necessarily in that order, but it is a reasonable one (tone examined before power testing may upset it ... sensation kept to the end because it's tricky and hopefully

---

[40] There was a test where you gently pressed the eyeball while fundoscopising, which normally makes the vessels at the disc 'pulsate', but doesn't in papilloedema. This has worked for me twice, but it's tricky to manipulate and there's an innate reluctance to press any eyeball but my own.

[41] If the examiner is not suitably astute, it may be stretching it to verbally suggest that you 'know the patient', hoping your embryonic relationship will allow them to agree. It does bring to mind the urban myth of the MRCP candidate who spent the night before the exam in the hosting ward, reading up all the case notes. Justice appeared to be served when his appointed case happened to be a new patient who had been brought in overnight. As he approached his quarry he stopped, told the organiser, 'I'm sorry, sir, I believe I've met this lady before'. He was commended on his honesty, and given another patient ...

[42] This advice is currently outdated, as the PACES exam system should result in your being given another fundus. However, I leave it as written since PACES itself shall surely perish as the tedium of examining on the same patient time after time provokes a revolt among the examiners who miss humiliating candidates on their pet cases (Mutiny of the Snickers).

the examiner will have got fed up and asked you to stop by then), and certainly you should stick to your own sequence – whatever it is – until it's slick. Neurological examination is classic for watching a candidate stutter through, continually wondering what to do next.

Tone

Don't check for it too rhythmically. Chop and change movements. It's often difficult to decide if tone is normal, and sometimes only the difference between left and right is clear. Classically UMN lesion (stroke, etc.) equals increased tone, and LMN lesion equals decreased tone. Recent UMN lesions, however, initially exhibit reduced tone (flaccid[43]), and since this gradually changes over time to increased tone, there must be a stage some time after a major stroke when the tone is normal!

Increased tone itself is usually categorised as 'spasticity' (UMN) or 'rigidity' (basal ganglia, e.g. parkinsonism). The former is classically described as 'clasp-knife', though a straw poll of colleagues reflected my own doubts that spasticity ever has this sudden release that everybody goes on about (indeed one suggestion was that the clasp-knife referred to the arm springing back into place when you tried to extend it) and which, to be honest, I more associate with feigned hypertonicity. The 'lead-pipe' sensation of rigidity I agree with, but spastic limbs are probably most often identified by the *degree* of hypertonicity, being potentially more severe than anything rigidity tends to produce.

It is also said that rigidity affects all muscles equally, spasticity having a predilection to anti-gravity muscles (witness the flexed-arm/extended-leg gait of an established stroke), but might this simply reflect the strength of the muscles?

The 'cog-wheel rigidity' of parkinsonism probably *is* the oft-cited mixture of lead-piping and tremor.

Power

Devise your own methods, working your way distally, and stick with them. 'Pronator drift' is a quick test for any mild weakness in the arm you may otherwise miss. The patient is asked to hold the arms outstretched, palms upwards. (**Accidental Contrariness No. 3** – they will always hold the palms down, even when you demonstrate … 'like this'.) Then you watch. If there is any weakness, slowly the hand will begin to drift … the ulnar side drops … the whole hand drifts down *and slightly out* …

Cynical Tip No. 20   If the patient is feigning weakness, the hand will probably drop *straight* down.

The legs have many muscle groups which you should not be able to overcome. For example, a patient digging their heels into the bed (gluteals) should be able to keep them there despite your best efforts. Anything less is weak.

---

[43] Pronunciation depends entirely on whether your senior colleague is male or female. With a male, use the 'X' sound in the middle.

> **Cynical Tip No. 21**   If the patient cannot raise their leg against gravity (i.e. against your hand resting purposefully on top of their leg but exerting no force) then they shouldn't be able to walk *at all* (i.e. if they walk into the consulting room and later cannot raise a leg …). But watch out for the effects of pain/discomfort.

Reflexes

Do learn the basic roots … which I really shouldn't lower myself to mentioning …
I mean, it's so … traditional …

Biceps	C**5**–6
Brachioradialis ('supinator')	C**5**–**6**
Triceps	C**7**–8
Knee	L**3**–4
Ankle	S**1**–2

Figures in bold are either all the more important or all the less important roots for that reflex. There, nobody's done that.[44]

- *Do* try to get the patient to relax the area you are testing – often by supporting it yourself.
- *Don't* break your back trying to support two huge legs so you can 'directly compare' knee jerks. Let your short-term memory take the strain. Chances are it's up to it.
- *Do* use the big lanky bendy tendon-hammer when available. (*Do not* be tempted to keep one in your pocket. Ophthalmologists make enough money as it is.) Tomahawks make it very difficult to perform the next tip …
- *Do* hit the tendon with a dead dunt. Reflex testing is the opposite of percussion of the chest where we wanted a quick bouncy flick on to pleximeter finger and back. The big lanky bendy tendon hammer is designed to deliver a dead thud. Don't go out of your way to try to stop it. It's amazing the number of students who percuss the way they should do reflexes and vice versa.
- *Do* use reinforcement when a reflex appears to be absent. The patient can either grit their teeth just before you 'strike', or clasp hands and pretend to pull them apart.
- *Do* know that this last procedure is called Jendrassik's manoeuvre.[45]
- *Maybe* recall vaguely that Jendrassik's manoeuvre works through gamma-motoneuron supply to muscle spindles increasing their sensitivity (*do* at least know that it's *not* just distracting the patient's attention).

Coordination

Basically, this is cerebellar function and not worth checking until you've confirmed that muscle power is fairly good. When doing finger–nose pointing, get the

---

[44] For why would anyone?
[45] Not to be confused with the *Dendrassi* – the race of aliens who cook for the Vogons … though again, why would anyone?

patient to 'stretch' slightly and move your finger just as they reach it. This helps to spot minor deficiencies, and is good fun[46] – particularly if you forget to mention at the start that this is your plan.[47] Don't be too quick to categorise poor-quality heel–shin[48] performances as within normal limits. Try it yourself and see how impressively perfect 'normal' is.

Dysdiadochokinesis. Take the patient through the manoeuvre stage by stage – 'building it up' – otherwise their blank look will be no more than you deserve.

Sensation

Proper examination of sensation – with the cotton wool and blunted sharp things (syringe needles jabbed repeatedly against the insides of their own casings; theoretically, otherwise they're too sharp to be painful!), etc. – takes for ever even without dashing off for test-tubes filled with warmish and coldish water.[49] The occasional patient coming up from Accident and Emergency with a straight line of pin-point bleeds stretching from ankle to groin has been enough to convince me that the elucidation of spinothalamic-ventroposterior nucleus connections is for someone who knows what they're doing and with some time on their hands. Sounds like a neurologist to me.

Simple sensation with light finger touch is worth taking time over, if it's part of the patient's complaint. Looking for root or peripheral nerve distributions. Patients find it easier to distinguish the change from paraesthesia to normal than the other way round, so moving your touch *out* of a patch of paraesthesia is usually best for defining areas. Maybe you should use cotton wool, but that just makes *me* uncertain whether the patient has been touched.

Cynical Tip No. 17 (addendum)   Hemi-anaesthesia/paraesthesia is unusual if not accompanied by other features. Assess it carefully (e.g. on the face with the eyes shut). The patient's pauses to think when they have nothing to think about may help, as may other occurrences. One patient who was admitted with left 'hemiparaesthesia', when asked to say 'fuzzy' or 'normal' as I lightly touched different parts of her face, got it consistently 'correct' until I touched her forehead in the midline. Pause ... 'can't tell – that's right in the middle,' she said. To which I innocently replied, 'That's OK. I was never asking you to tell me which side, just whether it's normal or fuzzy.' Eyes open. Pause again. I know. She knows I know. I know she knows ... We both know we can wait for it all to settle down without doing invasive tests or prescribing toxic therapies.

---

[46] Don't knock it. If grapes and water are available ...
[47] Do remember to emphasise that it is their own nose they will be touching. You don't really want a drunken lock-forward poking at your face.
[48] Note heel–shin. Not a vague splat of the foot moving down the leg. And get them to do it *slowly*.
[49] My favourite large textbook states 'Five primary sensory modalities – vibration, joint position, light touch, pinprick and temperature – are routinely tested in each limb ...' Aye right.

Financial Tip No. 1 (is this book comprehensive or what?) Do not take out critical illness insurance policies. Otherwise you will soon be struck down by an illness which does not quite qualify for payments (e.g. a hemiparesis which doesn't cause total loss of power in two total limbs totally). You may find yourself on the other side of the medical fence, massaging your symptoms and signs and *not getting better*. The other reason for not taking out such a policy is entirely superstitious. What would immediately happen if you ever cancelled it?

Proprioception in the big toe – remember to move the toe up and down with the fingers at the side (so the patient can't tell by feeling pressure, e.g. on the nail, that the toe is being pressed down). Normal proprioception can sense very small movements. Gross shoving around of the toe is not required (and is less discriminatory).

Cynical Tip No. 22 (not validated[50]) If the patient has supposed proprioceptive loss, but normal sensation otherwise, then doing this test 'badly' (i.e. pushing down on the nail) should enable them to tell which way it is going – and if they still can't ... ?

Cynical Tip No. 23 (validated[51]) Since they have a 50–50 choice, an anaesthetised monkey will get proprioception right half of the time, so a patient who consistently gets it wrong (rather than 'can't tell') is possibly feigning.

Vibrational sense
Seems straightforward, but I can't remember any instance when this gave me more information than proprioception (which tests the same 'dorsal columns' in the spinal chord). Normal patients often seem oddly unable to sense the vibration, even when the tuning fork is buzzed aggressively against their forehead or sternum as a demonstration. 'D'you feel THAT?!!!'

---

[50] Of course, none of the Cynical Tips are anything like 'validated', but this one is particularly theoretical. Even I don't believe it.
[51] See above. But ... this tip does appear in Hutcheson's *Textbook of Medicine*, so that does give it some more credence than my usual ravings.

Miscellaneous not necessarily useless information

Romberg's test

This is a test of proprioception (not cerebellum). You can stand up straight, feet together, with your eyes open, but with eyes shut you don't have the visual input to compensate for the lack of proprioception input and you sway and fall.

Dysphasia vs. dysarthria

It is easy to describe the difference, but not always to decide which condition the patient has. Dysphasia is a problem with the brain's formulation (expressive) and understanding (receptive) of language, mainly in Wernicke's area and Broca's area, respectively. Dysarthria is a problem with the articulation of speech. It follows correctly that dysarthria includes difficulty with speech because you have an ulcer on your tongue! Neurological causes of dysarthria include cerebellar dysfunction (described variously as 'scanning' or 'staccato' speech, despite these seeming obviously different), bulbar abnormalities (including UMN – 'pseudobulbar' palsy which can cause 'Donald Duck' or 'hot potato' speech; just because it's a UMN problem doesn't make it dysphasia) and basal ganglia problems. It really is difficult to tell one from the other by any of the standard descriptions or manoeuvres. I've asked 2000 patients to say 'British Constitution' (despite its being generally recognised that there is no such thing) without once being any the wiser.[52]

The rest of the signs will usually guide you.

An accompanying right[53] hemiparesis might help you to plump for dysphasia rather than dysarthria – the most likely level of distinguishing that will be required in an undergraduate exam. Other pointers to dysphasia include word substitution. Dysarthria is unlikely to make you say 'potato' instead of 'Gondolier'. Dysphasic subjects, on the other lighthouse, may do so. They may also 'explain' a concept. For example, if asked to name an object such as a pen,[54] they may get frustrated (another pointer to dysphasia?), saying '... *it's something you write with* ...', perhaps even managing '... *like a pencil* ...', saying these words perfectly well, but not succeeding in finding ... *'pen'*.

Dysphasia itself is usually mixed – not exclusively expressive or receptive – though ratios may vary. While examining, it is easy to persuade yourself that a dysphasia is purely expressive by giving subtle body-language hints of your requirements (e.g. 'raise your right arm in the air' said while raising your right arm

---

[52] Similar to the Babcock sentence which goes along the lines of 'one thing a nation needs to become both rich and great is a large secure supply of wood', and supposedly patients with early Alzheimer's can repeat it but not remember it. Neither can anyone else (hence the inaccuracy of my above attempt to remember it). Mainly because it's so stupid. You don't have to be reared on *Age of Empires* to realise that the country next door with the *metal* swords is 'gonna whup yo' ass!'

[53] I realise you all know that in right-handed people the language centre is in the dominant left hemisphere more than 90% of the time. In left-handers, it's about 50–50.

[54] This test of 'nominal' dysphasia is probably the most sensitive for picking up dysphasia. Making me always wonder if 'nominal' was subliminally suggesting that this was the mild version, as in 'nominal sum'.

in the air could gain an apparently appropriate response from someone with total aphasia,[55] as long as they otherwise have a few neurons to rub together).

Parkinsonism has a classic triad of *tremor* ('pill-rolling' = 3–5 Hz[56] – honest injun, seconds are *really* long things), *bradykinesia* (try asking them to take a pen from you) and *rigidity*. Remember that it usually begins *unilaterally*. That surprises a lot of people. Featureless features are a feature. The only thing to know about *glabellar tap* is that it's spelt with an 'a'.

Tremor deserves a pause. Parkinsonism is an example of *rest* tremor. Movement makes it less obvious. *Postural* (or positional) tremor is emphasised when the hand 'strikes a pose', as in the stretch your hands out to see if you're thyrotoxic (this very fine bilateral tremor just looks like nervous hands – only demonstrate it with the classic sheet of paper over the hands if the examiner is wearing a pinstripe suit). The *intention* tremor of cerebellar dysfunction is coarse and worsens uncontrollably as the hand nears its target.

Postural tremor is probably the most common, ranging from simple stress to the 'benign positional tremor' which appears as you get older and may run in families ('familial benign, etc ...'). The short-term benefit of alcohol is well recognised in the world of snooker.

Babinski response

The test is done by scraping a key or similar 'noxious stimulus' up the outer border of the sole of the foot and across the base of the toes. We are looking for the first movement at the first metatarso-phalangeal joint (big toe). It is normally downgoing, but in established UMN lesions the toe goes up (and, classically, the toes fan out as in babies). Since it is the first movement we seek, there is *no point* in continuing to scrape the *noxious stimulus* up and across the sole of the foot after we have seen the first movement. The outcome of the test will not be changed by any further movements – or screams – from the patient. In patients who withdraw, the stimulus may be made slightly less noxious by scraping up the outer border of the foot – not on the sole (*Chaddock's*). In fact there are countless ways of eliciting a positive Babinski. *Bing's* (giving multiple pinpricks on the dorsolateral surface of the foot) may be worth avoiding, but *Oppenheimer's* (pushing two fingers down the front of the shin) is worth doing as it looks cool, and sounds good.

---

[55] Total aphasia. A tautology (remember 'arrogant cardiologist'), since aphasia already suggests total loss as opposed to dysphasia. Or so I thought – apparently current psychology teaching has all of these as 'aphasia'.

[56] And I realise that you are familiar with the *hertz* unit of frequency, which essentially equals 'sec^{-1}' and has no connection with concepts of car hiring or one-born-every-minute.

6

Rheumatology

Rheumatologists are easy to categorise into two distinct types. Unfortunately, this can be done on at least three separate criteria.

By Method 1, Type A believes that rheumatology is the last bastion of general medicine. They revel in their position as one of a dying breed, practitioners knowledgeable in all fields. They nurture this belief in others and gaily take over the management of patients belonging to all and sundry at the slightest whiff of a rheumatological diagnosis – or simply because their diagnosis is regarded as 'tricky'. Type B takes the opposite view to the same scenario. They resent the imposition of constant requests to see (or even 'take over') everybody whose problem could conceivably include a rheumatological component. Patients with the worst illness on the planet, with the worst symptoms on the planet, eventually mention that their muscles ache, so the rheumatologist is dragged along and invited to take over the management of someone who should no more be under their care than a guy who's been impaled against a fence by a 10-inch spike through his thyroid should call an endocrinologist. While Type A demands to be informed of any patients with UTI/chest pain/pneumonia and an ESR above 42 in case they have SLE, Type B wants to be left alone to look after the people they think have arthritis (which is the disease they read about in a book once) and drink lots of good coffee (Type A likes instant).

Method 2 splits up rheumatologists into A – those who do pure rheumatology – and B – those whose jobs combine rheumatology and medicine. The pecking-order is nicely balanced. At meetings of Rheumatology Societies, those who also partake of the medical weed are rather frowned upon as 'jobbing' rheumatologists – enthusiastic amateurs whose superficial efforts are tolerated, but you wouldn't send your mother to see them. Much like your Rolls Royce and the local Kwikfit. Meanwhile, at gatherings of the General Medical Fraternity – including Scientific Academia – the jobbing rheumatologist has the upper hand, being at least seen as a *doctor*, while the pure rheumatologist is regarded as something of a rehabilitation super-physio.

Now, based on the above, you might expect there would be a tendency for the general physicians (Method 2) to be the ones who think that they're general physicians (Method 1), but oddly enough ...

The third method (Method 3) is scientific vs. clinical. I remember beginning a talk to students on SLE[1] with a vague (but beautifully delivered) vision of a multi-

---

[1] Bad syntax. You'll probably think SLE is a mind-altering substance ...

system disease which after 20 years I still didn't have a real handle on ... an eclectic mixture of apparently unconnected problems ... reflected in a research tool set of diagnostic criteria actually being used clinically ... The same talk, delivered to the next week's group by my colleague, began 'The Hep 2000 test differs from the double-stranded DNA antibody test in two crucial ways ... '

Again, it might surprise you that the dead-keen-for-lots-of-patients rheumatologist tends to be in the scientific group. Indeed, I now realise that all three techniques separate out the same groups. So we can amalgamate them:

- Type A: pure rheumatologists with a scientific bent who want every patient in the world to be considered rheumatological until proven otherwise.
- Type B: physicians with an interest who see quite enough patients thank you very much, like their coffee and shortbread and are entirely happy to leave the guy who fell off a roof and says his arm's sore ('Mr Smith wondered if it might be acute-onset rheumatoid') to the orthopods.

At our mythical cocktail party, Type B talks about things other than work, to save potential embarrassment. Meantime Type A, oblivious to reality, believes that being a rheumatologist is 'cool' and is happy to chat to all and sundry about cytokines and TNFα management policies on up-to-date analysis of bed distributions. All and sundry may not show the same enthusiasm.

Both types drive very ordinary cars, usually bought second-hand. Rheumatology is the converse of 'big earner' in the private world. Taking specialist and general history, doing specialist and general examination, and assessing the billions of specialist and general test results which rheumatology reliably produces, takes a long time. However, since these tests all go towards a huge bill from the labs and X-ray departments, the patient's only recourse is to give you the evil eye if you so much as ask for your own expenses. Unfortunately, unless you're an 'injector', the rheumatologist does not give the patient what they want – a quick diagnosis and a quick fix. Rheumatology Street in Private Medicine Land is not paved with gold. Rheumatologists therefore despise the cardiologist who spends two minutes confirming that the pain is in the patient's chest (and not someone else's) before performing and charging for an ECG, echo, angiogram/plasty – *then* saying they're OK. So much more persuasive than a few uncertain blood tests[2] and a lot of agonising. Chest pain sufferers who are told that they don't have coronary artery disease are usually relieved, joint pain sufferers who are told they don't have arthritis are usually unconvinced. And if the results *are* positive, would you rather pay to hear ' ... and this procedure should cure it ... ' or ' ... and if you take these tablets – and lots of other ones I'll tell you about as we go along (which will take some time because they've got oodles of side-effects) – for the rest of your life then we might perhaps maybe be able to get some sort of control ... '

So. If a second-hand Megane is your dream automobile ... read on.

---

[2] Perhaps X-rays are the answer. Patients believe X-rays can tell everything. Maybe we shouldn't correct their beliefs. 'Your X-rays look absolutely fine – so you're OK ... no, don't argue ... look! ... the X-rays are *normal* ... '

Rheumatology – history

Inflammatory arthritis

When seeing a rheumatology patient for the first time, the main question is 'Is this inflammatory arthritis or something else?', i.e. is this something which needs aggressive management with the triad of:

1   short-term symptomatic treatment
2   long-term disease control (DMARD[3] therapy)
3   joint protection measures

or something which needs a bit of general advice and monitoring?[4] Indeed, since (a) most rheumatology clinics' waiting-time for a routine appointment approaches one year and (b) proper inflammatory arthritis warrants the DMARD-type approach within 3–6 months (the delay being useful only in ensuring that it *is* rheumatoid arthritis and not, for example, some viral arthropathy), the process of weeding out the chaff from the wheat starts before you ever see the patient. Even from the GP's referral letter you must learn to pick up clues so that proper inflammatory arthritis gets seen more quickly than 'routine'. For simplicity's sake, let us call proper inflammatory arthritis 'rheumatoid'. Psoriatic arthritis, gout, reactive arthritis and others are all worth identifying, but rheumatoid arthritis (RA) is the one that patients have heard of, and it's the one they fear/desire.[5] And the quickest approach is to know – what rheumatoid arthritis *isn't*.

Rheumatoid arthritis isn't . . .
• Something which gives you pains all over your body.
• Something which you've had for 20 years without any visible damage to show for it.
• Something which gives you pains all over your body for 20 years without any visible damage to show for it.
• Something which, in the absence of any signs:
  – makes you drop things
  – makes your knee 'give way' when you're walking
  – makes you 'complain bitterly'[6] of pain.
• Pains which get worse at work or at night-time.
• An isolated positive rheumatoid factor.
• Something which starts off as a bad back.
• Something everybody must get if their mother or father was once told that *they* had it.

---

[3] Disease-modifying anti-rheumatic drugs – previously 'second-line' or 'slow-acting' drugs. When we realised that all proper inflammatory arthritis should be treated by these (since they prevent damage, whereas NSAIDs don't), the 'second-line' aspect was dropped.
[4] Connective tissue diseases and the like don't fit into this, but we'll get to that later.
[5] An odd juxtaposition, I admit. It is perhaps the 'label' of RA which some characters undoubtedly seek.
[6] Particularly useful in assessing GP letters. It's unclear whether the use of this phrase is a deliberate coded message from the practitioner, or simply his warding off future embarrassment. He justifies sending up someone who requires no rheumatological help by emphasising the patient's insistence.

Cynical Tip No. 24   A patient who has a family history of rheumatoid arthritis and attends your rheumatology clinic is *less* likely to have rheumatoid arthritis than someone who has no such family history. While there *is* a genetic component to the disease, the effect of this is far outweighed by the over-referral of patients with a family history whose personal story sounds no more like RA than Keifer Sutherland looks like an actor.

- Something which causes your ankle to be sore after you have fallen and twisted it and then when it fails to improve adequately under the ministrations of the orthopods you remember under close interrogation by said orthopods that you have had some pains in your finger (or 'generalised', as they will call it).

OK, it can be any of these, but usually:

Rheumatoid arthritis is ...
A variable, systemic disease. History of the joint component, however, comes down to three things. *1–2–3. Pain, Stiffness, Swelling.*

1   *Pain* should be in the joints. Not the muscles, bones, back, head ... the *joints*. If the patient has pains in the hands, ask them to point to which joints. In particular we're comparing MCPs vs. PIPs vs. DIPs.

Cynical Tip No. 25   Worth noting if they seem to resent this question.

---

2   Stiffness might be more vaguely situated.

> *1 + 2.* Both are worse in the morning.
> I'll say that again.
> *Both are worse in the morning.*
> If the pain is worse at night, it's almost certainly not RA (usually OA).

The duration of this 'morning stiffness' is also important, as any arthropathy (e.g. OA) will be worse for 10–20 minutes when you get up, but the 1 ... 3 ... 5 hours of severe stiffness very much suggests inflammatory arthropathy. Morning stiffness (or limbering-up time – LUT) is just *the* best question, though it can lead to interesting semantics:

> 'What time of day are your joints worst?'
> 'Every day.'
> 'But what time of day is the worst?'
> 'When I'm walking.'
> 'But what time of day?'
> 'What do you mean?'
> 'I mean, is there any time when they're always sorest, or extra stiff?'
> 'Nope ... the same all day.'
> 'So, no particular time ... like in the morning, or middle of the afternoon ...
>   last thing at night ... ?'

'Oh – in the morning ... they're definitely worst in the morning.'
'And how long does that extra worstness last for?'
'All day ... '

Cynical Tip No. 26 Non-steroidal anti-inflammatory drugs are very effective. They do exactly what they say on the tin. If the patient denies any help at all from these drugs, then the pains are *less* likely to be caused by inflammatory arthritis.

---

3   *Swelling.*   RA causes swelling of the joints. Real swelling. Not just something the patient describes as swelling. Including 'it looks OK but it feels swollen'.

Cynical Tip No 27   GP letters will often be very careful to say that the patient '... describes swelling ...' or '... complains of swelling ...' Assume that this means the GP has never seen this himself.

General puffiness over some vague area (usually the hand) is not necessarily joint swelling. Many patients will make much of the fact that they 'can't get their wedding ring on and off'. Most will happily reveal that they weighed 9 stones on their wedding day, but now tip the scales at around 15 stones (for those of you used to kilograms, that's a lot heavier than 9 stones). The idea that their hands may have become bigger will usually come as a shock. Try to find out if any *specific joints* have been swollen.

Cynical Tip No. 28   If the patient tells you that he or she gets swelling of the joints, but there is nothing to see at present ('this is a good day'), ask how long it tends to last for. The frequent answer of intermittent swelling lasting for a few hours at a time is not suggestive of RA.

Pain, stiffness and swelling. That's about it for deciding whether it's inflammatory arthropathy. What *type* of inflammatory arthropathy comes from other features – but before we discuss these, I should redress the balance of 'What rheumatoid arthritis isn't', since we can make mistakes in both directions.
Rheumatoid arthritis might be ... :

- innocuous arthritis – with MTP involvement
- innocuous arthritis – with MCP II and III involvement
- innocuous arthritis – with proper morning stiffness
- innocuous arthritis – in someone who never complains
- innocuous arthritis – with raised ESR, CRP or RF.

Any of these is enough to make you at least consider the diagnosis.

Other features

Onset

Take the patient through their story from the start. RA may have an insidious or a sudden onset, but the latter (anecdotally associated with a better prognosis) does raise other possibilities such as viral arthropathies or reactive arthritis. Note that these are separate diagnoses. There is a tendency among laymen (e.g. orthopods, GPs, professors of medicine) to use 'reactive arthritis' as a description of a viral arthritis. It is used more specifically by rheumatologists to describe an arthritis after (usually 1–3 weeks after) – for example – genito-urinary (*Chlamydia*) or gastro-intestinal (*Salmonella*, *Shigella*, *Yersinia*) infection, and occurs most commonly in patients who possess the HLA B27 antigen – the same genetic marker that is associated with ankylosing spondylitis.

Gout will usually present as a history of separate episodes of 1–2 joints being stupidly inflamed and sore and red and sore and untouchable and sore – this settling over a few days with anti-inflammatories. There does exist a 'palindromic rheumatism'[7] presentation of arthritis where the patient has a week or so of clearly inflammatory arthritis which settles, returning months or years later only to settle again, and this pattern repeats itself. Three things can happen to such patients. They may continue in this vein for ever, the problem may disappear, or it may drift into one of the conventional forms of arthritis ... the trick being to spot this last group early and treat them.

Events around the time of onset are worth eliciting. Viral symptoms may coincide with or precede onset. UTI or gastrointestinal upset may precede onset. RA itself may come on after any 'insult', such as bereavement, major illness, divorce or pregnancy – particularly the latter, since there is some unidentified 'protective' force in pregnancy which improves rheumatoid – leading to a higher incidence of onset after this period is over. As if someone was giving you steroids for no reason at all for nine months. When you stopped, if you'd had any onset of RA during that time, it would now present itself.

Distribution

Hands:

- *RA* – MCPs, PIPs
- *OA* – PIPs, DIPs, first CMC[8]
- *Psoriatic* – odd asymmetric mix of any of the above.

RA is hugely symmetrical. Small joints in the hands and feet are almost always involved – indeed the pain elicited on 'crunching' the MTP joints in the feet is often the single worrying feature on first examination.

Psoriatic arthritis is oddly asymmetrical – notably in the hands, where there may, for example, be a big swollen right index MCP, right pinkie PIP and left

---

[7] This name confused me for years. The palindromic ('Madam I'm Adam') analogy refers to the patient's returning entirely to normal after the event, so the episode of illness reads the same backwards ... as forwards ... apparently ...

[8] You won't know what this is. First carpo-metacarpal joint. Right down at the base of the thumb. If you've ever played *FIFA 2001/2/3/4/5ff* you'll know why it gets OA.

middle DIP in among a bunch of normal joints. The DIP is particularly useful, as it is simply *not* involved in RA (despite what some famous rheumatologist's might tell you).

Gout will classically start in the big toe (much more at MTP than in toe I-P joint itself) 50–75% of the time. The reason is unclear – but may be as simple as its obvious propensity to minor trauma. Recurrences can dot around the other joints.

Reactive arthritis will usually present as one or two large joints, usually of the lower limb, which are swollen (often remarkably so[9] – but not with the redness of gout) in a relatively young patient.

Viral arthritis will usually be of recent onset (after 3 months you start to think that something else is going on though it doesn't have to be). There is sudden onset, and it may have been accompanied by 'viral symptoms'.

History taking for specific areas

Tips – cynical and otherwise wise.

Hands
Find out where it's sore.

Cynical Tip No. 29   If the patient points vaguely to the dorsum or 'all over' the hand, it's not inflammatory arthritis.

Find out when it's sore.

Cynical Tip No. 30   Watch for an over-representation[10] of pains being worse at work – for example, ' ... when lifting things at work ...' ' ... while sitting at work ... '

Genuine work-related problems are usually relieved by time off work in the early days. As the disease progresses, the required lay-off time increases. Initially it'll settle by next morning, later it'll settle during the weekend, later still only if they have a week's holiday.

Shoulders
Ask about pain when brushing the hair – particularly in the morning.

Neck
Everybody has a sore neck. This is not suggestive of rheumatoid arthritis unless there are other pointers.

---

[9] My largest harvests (>300 ml) of fluid from aspiration of joints have all come from knees in reactive arthritis.
[10] Including one patient whose pains were worse when 'cycling to work', presumably as opposed to during other cycling.

Low back

Usually shunted by rheumatologists to orthopaedics (if this can be achieved – orthopods may not be the brightest stars in the Black Hole, but they are street-wise), unless it's the majorly-stiff-in-the-morning back of ankylosing spondylitis – usually starting in your twenties.

(Ridiculously) Heresy Tip No. 6   Back pain radiating down the outside of the leg as far as the ankle is usually fictitious (particularly if bilateral).   It just doesn't seem to follow a good enough nerve distribution for my liking. Others don't always agree.

Hips

Pains may be felt in various places. Usually outside of the hip or in the groin – but *possibly* behind the buttock, down the thigh, or even in the knee. These others, however, are usually associated with problems elsewhere, such as the back. Don't take a tale of 'hip pain' at face value. Nomenclature differs, as most patients have no idea where the hip is. A colleague refers to three types: (a) the 'proper' hip; (b) the *Marie-Claire* hip; (c) the *Country Life* hip (posh people can't say 'buttock'). Find out, sensitively, where it's actually sore.

Knees

Cynical Tip No. 31   Ask if the pain is worse when going up or down stairs – usually it should be worse (in the early days) going *downstairs*.

Ankles/feet

Cynical Tip No. 32   Pains all over the sole of the foot are not usually associated with arthritis, though patients may describe pains as all over the sole when they mean under the MTPs.

The classic feel of the metatarsalgia of inflammatory disease is like 'walking on pebbles'[11] or 'walking on glass'. If the earlier history has strongly suggested RA, you may wish to forego the benefits of not leading the witness and offer these descriptions to a patient who mentions foot pain – in order to impress them with your insight and knowledge.

---

[11] 'Pebbles' seems rather posh, but use of the vernacular can backfire. A Scottish east-coast physio colleague, used to referring to small stones as 'chuckies', told her Yorkshire class about this sensation of 'walking on chuckies'. Extremely odd looks and subsequent stilted rapport were only later explained when she found out that in that part of Yorkshire, 'chuckies' are chickens.

Non-inflammatory arthritis

Osteoarthritis

It's ... like ... wear and tear – innit? Pains in the joints gradually getting worse over the years but with occasional fairly sudden exacerbations (e.g. following viral insults, injuries, etc.). Patients will often discount the idea that they may have wear and tear since it all came on so suddenly out of the blue just months ago. However, careful history taking will reveal that either:

1   pains have actually, really, to be honest, when you think about it, been going on for some years *or*
2   'Out-of-the-blue' (OOTB) developed shortly after taking up horse riding or karate, or changing jobs from an accountant to being a trapeze artist (or vice versa) *or*
3   OOTB developed during and after a period of major weight gain *or*
4   OOTB developed some time after stopping being active (possibly with a brief trial at resuming activities to set things off) *or*
5   OOTB developed after some other insult, such as viral infection, bereavement, menopause, stopping HRT.[12]

Pains are often worse at night, and worse with (or after) exercise. They occur in sensible joints such as hips and knees. In the hands, the first carpo-metacarpal is classic. PIPs and DIPs develop hard swellings (Bouchard's and Heberden's nodes, respectively). Often these are very painful for the first 1–3 years while they are forming, and then the pain settles down.[13] The bumps remain and the mobility is hugely variable. Morning exacerbations last no more than 23 minutes. Osteo-arthritis can be really sore (that's why they replace hip joints!). Make sure that the patient realises that you realise this. When you diagnose wear and tear, that doesn't mean you think it isn't painful. Also reassure them that it doesn't just get worse and worse. People assume that 'degenerative' arthritis should do that, but it has good and bad spells like anything else.

Fibromyalgia

After an enduring phase of patients being 'upset' by this label, many now crave it – a marker for its increasing respectability. 'Fibromyalgia' began its days as 'fibrositis' – an artificial term[14] invented by GPs to explain inexplicable pains accompanied by fatigue. The alternative *'whingeing women syndrome'* (WWS – for it was indeed mainly women who suffered from this vague mixture of aches and pains) was too politically incorrect even in those days.

Years went by, and the aches and pains all over plus fatigue went in search of a real diagnosis. Since such patients attend different specialties depending on their situation and priorities, a number of new diseases arose:

---

[12] For some reason, many women develop joint pains when they stop HRT. Prominent at the time of writing when many have stopped abruptly because of worrying research findings. The effect may be a crystallisation of the previously uncertain observation of increased onset of pains at the menopause. Any explanation is complicated by the occasional pains after *starting* HRT which stop when the drug is stopped. Let's just put it all down to 'hormones' (*see* Chapter 9 on endocrinology).
[13] Confidently predicting this outlook for the patient, however, occasionally backfires.
[14] There was never any real suggestion that patients had inflammation of the fibrous tissue.

- *chronic fatigue syndrome* was diagnosed by psychiatrists/psychologists/GPs
- *post-viral syndrome* was diagnosed by infectious diseases specialists/GPs
- *benign myalgic encephalomyelitis* was diagnosed by a tiny subset of neurologists, but by 70% of journalists and *Sunday Mail* readers (who like to omit the 'benign')
- *fibromyalgia* was the preferred label for rheumatologists (though it needs be said that many persisted with WWS).

Features of the rheumatological version included the following:

- aches and pains
- fatigue
- morning stiffness
- poor sleep pattern
- irritable bowel syndrome
- paraesthesiae
- tender points.

However, the WWS tag was difficult to shake off. When you look at the list of symptoms it's easy to see why. Then someone looked at the EEGs of sufferers while they slept. This showed that they had less 'delta-wave' sleep (that deep fourth-level 'restorative' sleep that it takes some time to get into) than other people. This was assumed to be an epiphenomenon until some guy had the bright idea of stopping a bunch of super-fit American College Boys from getting their delta-wave sleep – and after a week of this they all got aches and pains and fatigue and morning stiffness and ...

This resulted in the suggestion that fibromyalgia was a 'sleep disorder', but the fallout from this revelation has been disappointing. Not so much that power-EEG analysis research has failed to come up with a cure, but more that rheumatology has failed to palm these patients off on some other specialty like sleepology. Clinics are still inundated with apprehensive/hopeful 'fibromyalgics'.[15] A clutch of fittingly vague criteria have been produced, namely:

- *widespread pain* (left plus right; upper plus lower limbs; plus back)

plus

- *tender points* ($>$10 out of 18).[16]

The latter are tested by pressing the points quite firmly, and seeing whether they are tender. Clearly not the most precise of tests. How hard is quite firmly? How tender is tender? The pressing should be at the firmness of blanching your own fingernail, but the tenderness ...? You can't really judge based on whether the patient says 'ouch' or 'ow', 'oya' or 'ssst'.[17] The tender points themselves are the nine bilateral points at:

---

[15] **Cynical Comment in Footnote No. 1** – even a vaguely understood label such as fibromyalgia is still a label, and as such helps subjects to obtain DHSS moneys, etc.

[16] This is always described as 11 or more out of 18, but I don't have a greater-than-or-equal-to sign on my keyboard, and this way saves all the words it would take to explain greater-than-or-equal-to. Always provided no footnote is required.

[17] For years I simply got the patient to say 'yes' or 'no' as I pressed the 18 points – occasionally accompanied by the odd 'ow!' or 'oya!'. Until one day, when I was examining a young woman with 'positive' findings, I was suddenly aware of how this might be sounding from outside the consulting room ...

Occiput	Back of neck, really
Low cervical	Either side of trachea
Trapezius	Top of mid-shoulder
Supraspinatus	Point of shoulder
Second rib	Medially, near sternum
Lateral epicondyle	About one inch distal to this
Gluteal	Gluteal
Greater trochanter	Anywhere round that area you didn't press for gluteal
Knee	Medial aspect.

These are areas of tenderness in many of us (for me it's the trapezius and low cervical), but we shouldn't have more than ten. Many practitioners such as myself use 'dummy points' – that is, pressing on other areas and seeing how the patient responds (there's no point in using tender points as a diagnostic test if the craziest person in the world with 18 positives is labelled fibromyalgia). This is frowned upon by fibromyalgia enthusiasts, but to me it makes the diagnosis much more convincing if someone has most of the 'correct' points tender and none of the dummies (I use dorsum of hand, mid forearm, shin, dorsum of foot, and skull).

If fibromyalgia is a sleep disorder, patients probably should have disordered sleep. Classically they have difficulty getting off to sleep, waken during the night and (importantly) have early-morning wakening around 5a.m. and can't get back to sleep. If the alarm wakes them every morning, they don't have this condition.

Hypermobility
Hypermobility syndrome consists of joint pains and evidence of lax ligaments. It is recognised as (1) causing aches and pains, (2) predisposing to injuries (sports, dancing, gymnastics – coaches hate prodigies having hypermobile joints that were able to do all the clever stretchy things before they were ever trained) and (3) predisposing to osteoarthritis in later life. It is *not* recognised as predisposing patients to (a) viral arthropathy with such organisms as erythro(parvo)virus B19 and (b) increasing pains in joints following less specific viruses. However, I strongly believe *that it does*.[18] Just because I am vilified at all rheumatological meetings as a crazy eccentric when I come up with this notion *does not mean that it isn't true* (that hypermobility predisposes to viral arthritic pains – *not* that I'm a crazy eccentric)!

Hypermobility is mainly diagnosed by examination – with a nine-point score consisting of:

1   pinkie (little finger) MCPs hyperextending to $90°$ ($\times 2$) (rest hand on a flat surface to examine for this; a hand in the air may *appear* to be this flexible)
2   thumbs hyperabducting[19] to touch the wrists ($\times 2$)
3   elbows hyperextending by $10°$ ($\times 2$)
4   knees hyperextending by $15°$ ($\times 2$)

---

[18] The concept first came to my mind during a minor 'epidemic' of parvovirus arthritis. The four consecutive young women I saw with the disease had 'coincidental' hypermobility.

[19] Defining 'hyper' varies between able to touch wrist, getting within a centimetre of wrist and getting parallel. The main thing to remember is for the patient to *hyperabduct* the thumb with gentle help from the other hand. They'll usually try to hyperextend the defenceless digit – and you should intervene *before* you hear any cracking sound.

plus the ninth point from the history – in their twenties, was the patient able to put entire hands flat on the floor when 'touching their toes'?

Four points out of nine plus joint pains equals hypermobility syndrome.

The significance of hypermobility is hotly debated. It is, after all, simply an extreme of normal – but once you look for it, it does appear to be the basis of many attendees at rheumatology clinics with non-specific joint pains.

It also probably predisposes to fibromyalgia, so you really must take it seriously ...

Examination

My local Med School is one of many to introduce the 'GALS'[20] system of rheumatological examination. This reminds the student to examine '**G**ait, **A**rms, **L**egs and **S**pine.' To this I would add '**C**omportment'[21] – the way the patient carries him- or herself, which you assess before you start the examination, even before you've taken the history. There's something about the way someone with pain moves which is very different from the way someone who wants you to think they have pain (or indeed, someone who thinks they have pain) moves.

GALS

Gait
Watch the patient. 'Antalgic gait' is an impressive phrase to use in an exam – but it simply means that the gait is an effort to avoid pain. To my mind, this describes every gait in the universe, including the normal (i.e. we don't walk about all day on our kneecaps). With years of experience, you'll learn to see from a patient's gait whether it's their hip or knee (or perhaps ankle) that troubles them. This will be more years' experience than I have, since I invariably get it wrong. Fortunately this talent is overrated since, if you wait a few seconds, the patient will usually tell you which bit's sore. More useful to a vet, really.

Cynical Tip No. 33 I remain aware that the patient is not aware of my incompetence in this area. Since it seems the sort of thing one *could* do, I might occasionally tell a patient who proffers an unconvincing story of knee pain that they walk as if it was the *hip* causing the bother (or vice versa). Then watch for the changes ...

Arms
Hands (real patients)
Observation: gently lift them up (one at a time is fine!) and look for swelling or discoloration over the joints. The joints that are affected give an idea of the

---

[20] GALS – Eastbourne burds.
[21] CGALS – Eastbourne birdies.

diagnosis. Look for deformity — but don't say this word out loud. Muscle wasting happens very quickly in arthritis — and is best seen in the hands at the first dorsal interosseus[22] muscle, which becomes flat, then concave.

Cynical Tip No. 34   If the patient flinches, moans and draws their hand sharply away when you gently lift it up — proceed with major caution. Either they have hugely tender arthritis, or — more likely since it is normal to avoid sudden movement of painful joints — no arthritis at all. Alternatively, you may have no knowledge of the word 'gently'.

Touch: feel the joints. Are any swellings warm, soft and tender (active inflammatory arthritis), or cool, hard and painless (osteoarthritis)? This is true for all joints — we're looking for extra warmth and swelling, and moving joints through range of movement (ROM) — so I'll not repeat it.

This next bit's good. You squeeze the joints. Doesn't sound like much, but it's about the only time as a doctor you get to deliberately cause pain.[23] Not only that, you can count up the pain and brag about it. Not needlessly, of course. There is a measurement of disease activity called the Ritchie Index.[24] A selection of joints in the body are 'pressed' and each is scored by the following format:

0   no pain
1   patient says 'pain'
2   patient says 'pain' and winces
3   patient says 'pain' and draws away (... slowly? ... see Cynical Tip No. 34)
4   patient doesn't let you touch joint in the first place.

The scores are then added together for an overall count. This can be used as a way of monitoring therapy and improvement (usually in research or audit), but isn't a part of normal examination. Its use has been largely superseded by other measures such as the DAS 28[25] (probably better, but much less fun).

---

[22] The dorsum of the web between thumb and index finger. Normally bulges when these fingers are clenched together, except in the aristocracy and female medical students.

[23] Opportunities to accidentally cause pain are, of course, legion. My favourite concerned a man brought to our Accident and Emergency following a heart attack. His GP had given him diamorphine which had been slightly over-effective. The patient was obviously in no distress, lying quietly with pinpoint pupils and breathing perhaps twice per minute. The opiate antagonist naloxone was clearly required and correctly given. The patient's response was instantaneous — immediately breathing normally, eyes wide alert ... and clutching his chest and screaming. My colleague murmured ' ... *intravenous pain* ... '

[24] Originating in Glasgow, this index enjoyed worldwide success and recognition, being the main index of activity in rheumatology papers for many years. When you read the technique described above, you will quickly realise that it was initially meant as a bit of fun rather than a world beater. This is reflected in the unheralded 'Ritchie' (an occupational therapist, I believe) being given first-author prominence (and subsequent immortality) in front of a clutch of rheumatological dignitaries who made up '*et al.*'.

[25] A composite score of swelling and tenderness in specific joints (guess how many) plus the ESR and a *visual analogue assessment of global activity* (that's marking a dot on a line which goes from 'feel absolutely brilliant' to 'feel absolutely minging' — very hi-tech).

The patient's power grip is then tested. You get them to grip your index and middle fingers (always two – they can hurt one or three, taking huge pleasure in doing so – no need to give them a chance to get their own back). To check the 'pincer' grip, ask the patient to pinch their thumb against each of the other fingers in turn.

Cynical Tip No. 35   Get used to normal hands. If the patient says that he or she has pains in the hands and they look and feel normal, they don't have inflammatory arthritis. There's also a characteristic stiff listlessness with which a hand with ersatz pain is held. Only learned by experience.

Hands are also assessed for the nail pitting and onycholysis (that funny nail raised from the nailbed looking like a fungal infection thing) associated with psoriasis/ psoriatic arthropathy.

This association is often confused. People with psoriasis may show these nail changes. If they do, they are more likely to have the arthropathy than other people with psoriasis – but they won't necessarily have it. Nothing stops people with psoriasis with/without nail changes from having osteoarthritis (a *very* common disease) or RA – so the presence of psoriasis or nail changes *does not turn barn-door OA into psoriatic arthritis.*[26] Meantime, psoriasis may run in families, along with psoriatic arthropathy, some members getting both, some neither and some one or the other. You may have psoriatic arthropathy and not have psoriasis! Psoriatic arthritis can occasionally produce 'dactylitis' – a sausage-shaped finger (or toe) in which all the joints and intervening tissue appear to be homogenously swollen and often discoloured.[27]

Limited joint mobility (LJM) is a relatively common finding in patients with diabetes. They are unable to fully extend the fingers, this being demonstrated by asking them to 'say their prayers' (with the minimum of menace), whereupon they are unable to put the fingers flush against each other. Oddly, this sign (along with Dupuytren's) has been shown to be strongly associated with the vascular complications of diabetes such as retinopathy. LJM itself may thus be a manifestation of small-vessel disease. While originally termed 'cheiroarthropathy', this description has been dropped as it has nothing to do with the joints and isn't painful. It should not be confused with arthritis.

Carpal tunnel syndrome can occur in RA. It causes pain/paraesthesia in the distribution of the median nerve's $3\frac{1}{2}$ fingers. Tingling in all of the fingers doesn't suggest this. Normal thumb and pinkie, but other fingers all affected, is another favourite of patients without carpal tunnel syndrome. Tapping over the radial aspect of the front of the wrist (Tinel's sign) may induce the symptoms, as may holding the patient's wrist in forced flexion for up to 30 seconds (Phalen's). Abduction of the thumb is supplied by the median nerve alone, and a weakness in this movement is a more serious sign. Unfortunately, it takes three hours to get the patient to hold their hand out, palm up, and try to move their thumb up

---

[26] Unless you're an orthopaedic surgeon who wants to fob off your patient on to someone else's list.
[27] General tendinitis may be the explanation. Doesn't explain why we can spell tendonitis with an *i*.

towards their nose while you try to prevent this, so you may have to use opposition of the thumb with pinkie (includes ulnar input) as a surrogate.

Hands (exams)

Now.

All of the above concerns real patients − working out what's wrong with them so we can make them better, and that sort of stuff.

This has no relevance to clinical exams.

Examiners know almost nothing about rheumatology. It's a law. They only know three things: (1) ulnar deviation, (2) swan-neck deformity and (3) buttonhole (Boutonnière) deformity.

1   They will neither know nor care why the fingers deviate in the ulnar rather than radial direction (nor, if you pressure them, will they be entirely convincing as to which is which), but will feign a major interest in having your opinion. The normal argument is that it's simply due to the effect of gravity. My own view is that it's an exaggeration of the normal drift you see when you clench your fingers − so the shape of the ligaments/joints already allows for it.

2 + 3   Swan-necking and Boutonnière are shown in the following figures. Learn which one is which − even though this is of no consequence. If you do forget (a list of two is always the hardest), don't panic. A bit of confidence should

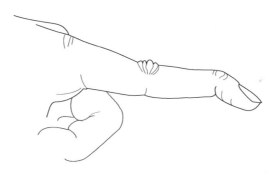

Swan-necking

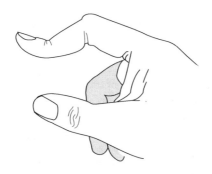

Boutonnière

bluff them, and since no one knows why they happen, the conversation is likely to revolve around whether it's supposed to look like a buttonhole[28] or a buttonhook and what the hell a buttonhook[29] is, or indeed was, anyway.

Learn these for the exam, then forget them … until you yourself are examining in the future. The other thing to remember for exams is to examine the elbow 'as part of the examination of the hands' (don't let the facts get in the way of good technique) for the nodules of RA (which means that the diagnosis is *as good as made*) or evidence of psoriasis (which *doesn't*).

Exam Tip No. 2   Spend time practising saying 'metacarpophalangeal joints', 'proximal interphalangeal joints' and 'distal interphalangeal joints' out loud in a closed room. The first time you describe the MCPs, PIPs and DIPs in any exam, use the full name fluently, falling back on the abbreviations from then on.

Rest of arms
See if the wrists or elbows are warm or swollen. Bend the elbows and 'rotate the wrists'. See if they are sore.

Cynical Tip No. 36   'Rotating the wrists' mainly rotates the elbow, and shouldn't really cause much wrist pain. The wrist will only do its 20–30° if you fix the forearm.

Shoulders
Ask the patient to put their hands behind the back of their head, then to put their hands behind the back of their back. If they manage that OK, the shoulders are pretty much OK. If they don't, then there's lots of really complicated details about rotator cuffs, painful arcs (do it yourself – bring your outstretched arm, palm facing outwards, slowly down from upright. It's sore at around 90°, then gets better) and stuff that suggest problems outside the joint ('impingement' and the like[30]). Meanwhile, rotating an arm hanging down at the side but bent at the elbow actually checks the shoulder (gleno-humeral) joint itself. But we shouldn't get involved with all that because:

---

[28] Either the hole that a button goes through or the flower on a wedding lapel. You'd think these were so different that it's obvious which is referred to. But no. An alternative suggestion is that it resembles a finger that has been stuck through a buttonhole … but … why?

[29] Rather like the 'Waterhammer pulse' description of the collapsing pulse of aortic incompetence. A ubiquitous footnote would describe this 'Victorian toy' as a large tube with water in it. You turned it over and … er … the water went down to the other side. Supposed to help one recognise the clinical abnormality, this reference served only to convince me that the Victorians were much more easily 'amused' than M'Lady's famous quote had led us to believe.

[30] I've recently been won over by an alternative impingement test (Hawkin's). Arm pointing straight forward from the shoulder, elbow bent at 90° so forearm goes across face … rotate hand down to point to floor – ouch!

1   I never did get the hang of it
2   much of it was worked out by orthopods, and since they're only looking for an excuse to stick needles into things before chopping said things out, then referring them to rheumatology when they're not cured, we can't really trust them (what, exactly, gets ... impinged ... on to ... what?)
3   somebody published a paper recently comparing the results of all these tests with MRI scans showing what was really wrong – the correlation was abysmal (*see* point 2).

Legs
Straight leg raising (SLR) is really a check of the back. If it is painless to $> 80°$ there is unlikely to be any major lumbo-sacral problem.

Cynical Tip No 37   Back/back-of-leg pain is unlikely before raising the leg by 40°. If it occurs, then later try sitting the patient *upright* with their legs *straight out* in front of them while you 'press the spinal processes'. This may well be revealingly pain-free if the patient fails to spot the familiarity of the manoeuvre (they don't have the italics to help them). Occasionally, pressing the spinal processes might be sore – for no particular reason that I can make out.[31]

Hips
'Rolling' the straight legs on the couch is a gentle test of the hips, but it is more sensitive at picking up hip problems if you bend the knee and then rotate the hip.

Bending the knee and pushing it up towards the contralateral shoulder checks for sacro-iliitis on the side of the leg.[32] Again there is a more sensitive test. Budge the patient, lying on their back, across the couch and pull the near-side leg over the edge and down towards the floor. Don't let them topple over.

Cynical Tip No. 38   In anyone who has nothing wrong with their joints, but wishes you to think that they have, all of this energetic testing of the hip will cause pain in the *knee*. So don't tell them you're checking the hips.[33]

Knees
Observation: The best place to look for muscle wasting is the *vastus medialis* part of the 'quads'. It doesn't atrophy any faster than anything else – it's just more obvious.

---

[31] A 'gentle thumping' down the spine is a recognised part of rheumatological examination. I'm not sure what rheumatological condition causes this to be painful. Maybe osteoporotic fractures. Maybe sepsis in bone. Arguably neither rheumatological.
[32] You're not expecting it to reach the shoulder – but it helps that they don't know that (see below).
[33] It's a bit like being a magician. Both in the principle of 'misdirection' and in not letting the audience know in advance the effect of a trick. Particularly with card tricks, people don't notice that a magician rarely tells you at the start what effect he plans to achieve – so you don't watch for the right things.

Examination: Just put your hand on it and wobble it about.

• Warm boggy swelling at the knee is the same as that at any other joint.
• Range of movement should go well past 90°.
• Laxity of collateral ligaments is tested with the knee relaxed and slightly flexed (as the quadriceps would otherwise keep the knee stable).
• Cruciates testing does *not* require you to sit on the patient's foot. Presumably this technique was invented by a one-armed orthopod.
• Crepitus is a nice crackling feel under your hand. It's a sign of OA and should be present in any self-respecting male over the age of 50 years.

Which brings us to:

Effusion: Lots of guff has been written and spoken about examining for knee effusions. Essentially you'll very quickly get used to the feel of the knee, learn to wobble the patella about a bit and know whether there's fluid there. (Though occasionally florid synovial hypertrophy can deceive you – causing major embarrassment at the subsequent aspiration of next to no fluid in front of an enthusiastic group of students). However, for clinical exams there's an obligatory routine of squeezing fluid down from the suprapatellar pouch, then either tapping the patella against ... whatever it is underneath ... or brushing your finger delicately down one side of the knee to demonstrate a bulge appearing on the other side ...

I suppose the thing to do is just feel the knee, decide if there's fluid ... then manipulate these tests (as they can be manipulated) to 'show the examiner' whether or not there is fluid there.[34]

Ankles
Remember that lots of patients think that oedema is a swollen ankle ... and that this will therefore be painful. So do some GPs.

Feet
Brilliant test. You crunch the MTPs between your fingers and thumb, pressing sideways from big toe through to little toe. *Any* inflammation (RA, classically) and this will be very painful. Often they will jump and you can raise a smile by asking them 'Was that sore at all?' It is usually accompanied by the 'walking-on-pebbles' history. Often an entirely normal clinical examination with all the hallmarks of 'mild osteoarthritis' will be turned on its head by the finding of general metatarsalgia. Even on its own, this sign must make you consider inflammatory arthritis – particularly RA.

Spine
According to an old boss, any rheumatologist who is planning to take himself seriously requires a goniometer to examine the spine. It is a deceptively complicated device with wires and things and a meter which measures degrees. Why make vague estimates of spinal ROM when you can actually measure it accurately?

---

[34] This shouldn't be a high-risk strategy. The person who decided for the examiners whether there is an effusion presumably knew what they were doing, wobbled the patella and came up with the same answer as yourself. It's unlikely that the examiner will produce an X-ray, or ultrasound (or big white needle!) to prove you wrong.

Never used one, myself.

Bought a tape-measure instead.

Basically, when it comes to the spine and rheumatology, we're talking ankylosing spondylitis. Everything else is orthopaedic (?!) So, how stiff is the spine? Wall-to-tragus is the boys. You put heels against the wall, buttocks against the wall, and try to put your head (the back of it) against the wall. If you succeed, all is well (and the wall-to-tragus distance will be around 12 cm). If you fail, the WTT will give a measurement of how badly, and this can be monitored over the years.

The other best quick spinal test is of lateral flexion. The upright patient tries to put the flat of his right hand down past the outside of his right knee (this being the level of 'OK').

Yet another best test for ankylosing spondylitis was mentioned in an earlier chapter,[35] namely chest expansion. The tape measure is held all the way round the chest − taut − while the patient breathes all the way out. Then they breathe in and you see how much the chest expands. The normal distance is 5 cm, but for some reason anything over 3 cm is conventionally accepted as satisfactory.

Sacroiliitis[36] we tested with the legs, though it is really a part of spinal examination (as indeed is SLR). It's easier for patients if you examine things while you're there, rather than going through system plans − making them sit up, lie down, sit up again, roll over on to your left, now right, now left …

Neck

Should have mentioned this really. Do it while you're 'doing' the shoulders. You gently lead the patient's neck through the six movements: flexion (chin should reach chest); extension; left and right rotation; left and right flexion. These last are the most sensitive and should cause some pain if there are any decent problems in the cervical spine − including simple cervical spondylosis. There's a story that all six movements are never painful except in the rare occurrence of malignancy. Not validated enough to be a Cynical Tip (?!), but I have noticed that most patients who purport to experience pain on all six movements have little else to suggest organic disease.[37]

A general rheumatological examination will also include:

1   a look for any odd rashes − including the butterfly rash of SLE, the erythema nodosum of sarcoidosis,[38] and the unusual 'livido reticularis' associated non-specifically with anti-phospholipid syndrome

---

[35] Though I did get rather bogged down in a metaphysical discussion of the mysterious interrelationships of the numbers 5 and 2.

[36] It's possible betting money can be won on this as an example of a word with two consecutive *is*. It's also possible some money can be made on a sentence such as that last one that ends correctly with '*is*'. Just possible, that is.

[37] And if so, this wouldn't be the first sign to suggest it's either (a) malignancy or (b) nothing wrong with you.

[38] The classic presentation of sarcoid in a young woman is erythema nodosum plus ankle arthritis. A chest X-ray with bilateral hilar lymphadenopathy should confirm the diagnosis. This is often self-limiting (though it may require steroids and/or bed rest to help it along) and non-recurring. The other presentations of this bizarre systemic granulomatous disease are not usually so benign.

2   an entertaining squeezing of all the main muscle groups (in the limbs). Proximal tenderness may suggest either polymyalgia rheumatica or the more worrying myopathy/myositis problems such as polymyositis. Distal tenderness may suggest no such thing (though it can occur with vitamin D deficiency, or 'inclusion body myositis')

3   pressing of tender points (*see* Fibromyalgia).

Specific diagnoses

There are one or two rheumatological diseases which require separate consideration.

Gout

Big red hot swollen painful tender joints which last a few days, and settle with anti-inflammatories. Usually gout starts in the big toe (not actually *in* the big toe but at the metatarso-phalangeal joint), but sporadically goes on to involve other joints in later episodes. If left alone, it may become grumbling chronic.

The erythema may move along the limb away from the joint (e.g. at first MTP going along the medial border of the foot), raising the possibility of an alternative diagnosis — cellulitis. Moving the joint 'from a distance' (i.e. without touching the red bit) may help distinguish these. Almost pain-free in cellulitis, this should still cause gratifying agony in gout.

Tophi may occur in the upper border of the auricle (the big floppy part of the ear), and finding these may obviate the need for joint aspiration to confirm the diagnosis. Otherwise rheumatologists swear by the finding of strongly negatively birefringent crystals under polarising microscopy before starting long-term therapy with allopurinol. Patients with uncertain diagnoses are told to turn up at short notice if they have a flare. The joint can then be aspirated and the diagnosis 'proven'. Being aware of the excruciation I cause when sticking a needle into a huge tiny big toe joint, I usually suggest that they turn up the first time it affects the knee ...

Polymyalgia rheumatica

History: Old person. Aches and pains in proximal muscles (over shoulders and hips/ thighs). Worse in the morning. Stiff, extremely so in the morning. Off food. Depressed. Can't be bothered. Grumpy.

Examination: Can't be bothered. Grumpy. Tender over upper arms and thighs (may jump!).

Blood tests usually show a rise in inflammatory markers — possibly huge (try all of them — ESR, CRP, immunoglobulins and plasma viscosity) with normocytic anaemia.

Responds like *magic* to 15 mg prednisolone, usually within 72 hours, and certainly within a week. This can pretty much be used as a diagnostic test in uncertain cases[39] (e.g. with normal blood tests). If it fails to make an impression after one week, *stop it* and consider other possibilities.

---

[39] Note that the diagnostic test is 15 mg prednisolone. The old-fashioned (unfortunately still seen) use of 60 mg prednisolone would make you feel better during a plane crash.

If the ESR, etc. *are* high, but the response to prednisolone is unimpressive, consider atrial myxoma and renal tumour. They do happen.

Temporal arteritis

Associated with PMR. Either may occur in isolation, but PMR is much more common. Again, the patient is often miserable, grumpy, off their food, usually with aches plus ... headache – usually over the temporal artery.[40]

Clinical findings over the artery are often misunderstood. It is *normal* to be able to feel the pulse, and this may be lost in temporal arteritis. It is *not normal* to be able to feel the vessel itself, and this may be *present* in TA.[41]

ESR should be hugely raised, but we never say 'always' in medicine either.

Vitamin D deficiency (osteomalacia)

This causes pains in the muscles, bones, joints ... everywhere. It is quite common in my clinic, as osteomalacia is *designed* to affect local Asian women. I'll explain. You get vitamin D from two sources – diet and sun-induced synthesis in the skin.

1   Phytates in chapatti flour bind to vitamin D in the diet and prevent its absorption.
2   Dark skin reduces the effect of the sun.
3   Customary clothing may mean that most of the skin is covered most of the time – reducing the effect of the sun.
4   They are in *Glasgow* ...

It is important to consider vitamin D deficiency – if only because it is so easily treated. Bone metabolism experts will go into lots of details about its diagnosis (does it *really* require a bone biopsy?), but most rheumatologists are happy to treat any vague pains accompanied by low blood levels with calcium and vitamin D preparations and see what happens.

Connective tissue diseases

The bane of the rheumatologist's life, and yet the excitement. A huge spectrum of disease ranging from vague aches and pains to catastrophic multi-organ failure, itself varying from shockingly acute to relentlessly chronic. All vaguely connected by the presence of funny antibodies to your own cells, nuclei, bits of nuclei ...

Explaining CTD to a patient is like explaining the origins of the universe to your son who wants a space-suit. Once you've bought him the suit, he's then at the level of a doctor trying to understand CTDs. They're not easy.

The thematic diagnosis is systemic lupus erythematosus (SLE). You can tell a disease is difficult when a set of research-orientated criteria is used in the clinical setting. Such criteria are produced so that researchers across the world know (or

---

[40] An apparently obvious point happily ignored by those keen for rheumatologists to do their work for them.
[41] Owing to a last-minute change in chapter order, this concept has already been repeated ('iterated').

can pretend) that they are talking about the same group of people when comparing such things as natural history and new therapies. The criteria are not really meant for clinical use. Otherwise invoking the criteria for *possible, probable* and *definite* rheumatoid arthritis – which include such things as:

- swelling in a joint
- swelling in a joint seen by a doctor
- swelling in another joint ...

would bring your clinic to a standstill. With SLE, however, the nebulous nature of the disease itself has reduced us to using the following criteria:

1   butterfly rash
2   discoid lupus erythematosus
3   mouth ulcers
4   photosensitivity
5   non-destructive polyarthritis
6   serositis
7   'cerebral lupus'
8   haematological disorder (thrombocytopaenia, leucopaenia ...)
9   immunopathological disorder (LE cells, anti-DNA antibody ...)
10 renal disease (proteinuria, casts ...)
11 positive anti-nuclear antibody (ANA).

Any four of these theoretically 'makes' the diagnosis of SLE.[42] Two features which have been 'dropped' from the original diagnostic criteria are actually much more fun. They are sorely missed, particularly since the new arrangements leave two immunological criteria essentially saying the same thing, presumably to please the scientists. Raynaud's phenomenon was felt to be so common that it wasn't discriminatory. I should clarify here that Raynaud's occurs when hands or part of the hands go *white* in the cold. Not *blue* – nor indeed *stiff*. This is painful. On returning to warmth they usually go through another colour phase (e.g. purple – again usually painful or at least itchy) before returning to normal.

Cynical Tip No. 39   If you just ask patients if their hands do anything funny in the cold and they don't come up with a good Raynaud's story (i.e. *you* have to explain it to *them* before they agree), they don't have Raynaud's phenomenon.

The other hero not required for the big match is alopecia. It's to be noted that the problem associated with CTDs is at the level of bald patches. Not thinning. *All* women of a certain age,[43] if asked whether their hair is falling out will say 'yes.' It's as if no one ever told them that hair is constantly growing and falling

---

[42] Again, people will have SLE who do not fulfil the criteria – and vice versa (you know what I mean). It is a research tool to enable populations to be studied – but it's also the best we've got clinically.
[43] I have no particular age in mind. I introduced the phrase only on realising how misogynistically the sentence read otherwise.

out. Every time they wash it and find some hairs in the plughole it comes as a new surprise.[44]

Other features to note on specific criteria include the following:

1   Butterfly rash is a bit like malar facies but looks as if would glow in the dark. Linked to 4.
2   DLE is a dermatological diagnosis. The main thing to know is that DLE plus aches and pains does not necessarily equal SLE. Let them keep attending the dermatologists.
3   Mouth ulcers are like usual simple aphthous ulcers – just more than normal. I usually use this opportunity to ask about genital ulcers, a symptom of the rare Behçet's disease.
4   Photosensitivity. A skin thing. *Not* headache or eye strain or nausea in the sun. Nor is it blistering after lying on a Majorca beach for 12 hours. Any rash in Scottish sunshine is, on the other hand, pathological.
5   Terrible pains in the joints with nothing to be seen can be nothing at all, but can be SLE.
6   Unexplained pleuritis, pericarditis or peritonitis.
7   Can be at the level of seizures or cranial nerve palsies or psychosis – but could the apparent increase in 'odd personality' in SLE be a minor manifestation of cerebral lupus?[45]

So the 'connective tissue enquiry' asks about Raynaud's phenomenon, alopecia, aphthous ulcers and photosensitivity as above ... and also about the eyes (dry/ gritty with regard to Sjögren's[46]), swallowing (poor oesophageal peristalsis in scleroderma – the sticking of food usually occurs at the sternal level, not in the throat) and any odd rashes (dermatomyositis, anti-phospholipid syndrome[47] ...).

Some CTD patients lend themselves to confident diagnoses. Most, however, defy any precise classification. Even if you're sure they've got a CTD, it won't be clear which one. They all merge together, despite measurement of the various auto-antibodies – which are an absolute minefield to a sensible person.[48]

But does this make them the bane of a rheumatologist's life? Yes. Not only are they difficult to diagnose precisely, and not only are they potentially very dangerous, but they are also a useful 'likely diagnosis' for a non-rheumatologist to make in *anyone* who is a diagnostic puzzle. And once someone is labelled 'query CTD' and sent along to you, it's very difficult to exclude it and send them straight back again.

---

[44] Since we're on a misogynistic footnote theme, I'll compare this to the surprise experienced by females when they eventually get to the front of queues (e.g. in the canteen) and apparently discover that they actually have to pay for their selections ... so *then* they hunt for their purse ...

[45] The occurrence of odd personality with the disparate symptoms of SLE can make the disease difficult to distinguish from ... odd personality.

[46] Schirmer's test is a nice technique that involves hooking a sliver of sterile filter paper on to the patient's eyelid and seeing if it wets down 10 mm in 3 minutes, or 15 mm in 5 minutes, depending on which book you read. I tend towards the shorter version – and anything under 10 mm but over 5 mm I wouldn't jump to call abnormal. A darkened room may ease discomfort (but not so dark you accidentally poke an eye with your thumb).

[47] You may have noticed this disease cropping up repeatedly with no explanation of its nature. I'm trying to re-create the effect 'SLE' had on myself and colleagues in *our* young days.

[48] There is even an official antibody – anti-RNP – which is specific for 'mixed connective tissue disease'. Enough said.

7

Gerontology

This specialty's inability to take itself seriously is reflected in its inability to find a title that it's comfortable with.

Geriatrics was discarded because many practitioners resented being a 'geriatric consultant'.

Gerontology was toyed with, as it made their discipline sound much more scientific. However, this was dismissed as inappropriate for exactly that reason.

The preferred title now depends on which part of the country you are visiting. Scotland goes for variations of *Medicine for the Elderly*. However, the acronym 'ME' has all the wrong connotations, being the title of a disease the existence of which most practitioners totally fail to believe in.[1] Many therefore used the *Department of Medicine for the Elderly* acronym of DoME. However, the insistence of a number of my colleagues (OK – me) on pronouncing this as 'Dommy' (as in 'domiciliary visit' – the very sort of thing that the geriatricians were trying to shake off[2]) soon got them to drop the 'o' and simply describe their specialty as *DME*. This does lead to a slight discrepancy, since while others will describe their specialty as psychiatry or orthopaedics, the geriatricians' 'specialty' is *DME*. A bit like someone at our cocktail party introducing himself as 'an Institute of Neurological Sciences'.

England is more keen on *Care of the Elderly* variants – apparently oblivious of the fact that this suggests no need for their subjects to be ill in any way. Maybe they go round and make any retired couples in their catchment area a nice hot dinner before they go off to the bowling or a Rotary Club meeting. Such drawbacks are likely ignored, however, as the phrase *C of E* probably gives them a comforting sense of security.

Northern Scotland experts go for 'Healthy Ageing' (or something) which seems fine for a herbal remedy shop, but not exactly a career for someone with a medical degree.

Geriatric consultants at our cocktail party *do* have a consistent title. They are called gatecrashers.

Geriatric consultants don't drive cars, as it's illegal – in case they fall asleep at the wheel.

Gerontological history

Ask the patient how old they are.

---

[1] I know. Don't end a sentence with a preposition – but you just try putting that last thought (plus subtext) together without breaking at least one rule of syntax that we should all be trying to keep to.
[2] I know.

Cynical Tip No. 40   Don't believe the females.

Also ask them how many stairs there are in/up to their home.[3]

Gerontological examination

Take the patient's pulse and ask them to say 'aaaah'.[4]

---

[3] **Ageist Tip No. 1**. These figures may be added to give the Geriatric Living Index of Mobility Problems in the Social Environment (GLIMPSE). Anything over 90 is 'vulnerable'. Doesn't give the whole picture, but ...

[4] For a really professional touch, look in their mouth using a pen-torch while they're doing this.

8

Alternative medicine

'Alternative medicine' is a misnomer – since any respectable practitioner will usually encourage the presence of conventional medicine in the background.[1] The term 'adjunctive medicine' is, however, ugly and unhelpful, and after years of suggestions (holistic, natural, complementary ...[2,3]) the term 'alternative' has rather stuck for the lack of a clear ... alternative.

The main thing to know about AM is that you're not allowed to say it's absolute rubbish, but neither are you allowed to espouse it with any enthusiasm. The medical establishment is, as mentioned, extremely conservative. But it is also extremely timid. It tries to keep in with everyone. Thus while it may be convinced that homeopathy (just to pick an example from thin air – rather in the manner that homeopathy was) is absolute tommyrot, it is afraid to use such offensive terms in public.[4] The press would be quick to take the opposing view, quoting the more reasonably stated cases of proponents – 'we shouldn't be dogmatic ...' and 'everything should be looked into ...'[5]

It's a clever ploy, when championing something outrageous that flies in the face of current knowledge, to take a very reasonable, almost uncertain stance. That way any robust defence from the establishment will make them look like the extremists.[6] Meantime, the alternative riposte – an equally reasonable approach admitting the possibility that these things *may* work – unfortunately gives many of these disciplines a credibility they hardly merit (as did the use of 'disciplines'). We must feel for these poor Establishment chappies (honest) – caught in the horns of a dilemma. Look like an extremist (and possibly lose out on some Royal patronage[7]) or admit the possibility of something being useful when you are convinced it isn't.

We don't know everything – but that doesn't necessarily mean anybody can say anything and it must be taken seriously. We do well to admit, however, that the

---

[1] Including to avoid being sued if real disease fails to respond to alternative remedies.

[2] 'Complementary' may well be the best term, though ingénue patients might assume it'll be free.

[3] In fact, I swithered over calling the chapter 'Complementary medicine'. On consulting Google, AM got 16 000 000 hits while CM got 4 000 000 hits, so I've stuck with the former.

[4] Their idea of an offensive word being 'tommyrot'.

[5] I made these quotations up. But today's newspaper carries a letter from a local homeopathy fan reminding us that 'it is important to have an open mind'.

[6] This is now technically termed 'being defensive', and for some reason which continues to escape me, this 'being defensive' – which apparently consists of arguing your case by giving examples and using logic – is evil and a sure sign of being wrong.

[7] The enthusiasm of certain members of the Royal household for AM is well known. It adds to its credibility. The public apparently considers that having the Queen as a relative establishes one's credentials for deciding what medicines people should take. Would they let HRH write and install a virus scan on their computer?

world is forever changing. Years ago in a society dominated by religious, voodoo-esque or other witch-doctory, the use of an extract of foxglove for swollen ankles would probably have been considered worse than 'alternative'.[8] We must remember this before we dismiss AM as the nonsense it almost universally may be ...

Herbal medicine

Clearly the healing powers of herbal remedies cannot be discounted. What are digoxin, atropine and aspirin if not concentrated extracts (sort of) from foxglove, deadly nightshade and willow bark? The only bogus feature of herbal remedies' promotion is any assertion that they are totally safe and cannot cause side-effects. They are untested, irregularly dosaged, potentially active/toxic materials and as such must be viewed with some caution. Something like old wives themselves. Remember to ask patients if they're taking any herbal remedies. Some can cause toxicity while others, such as St John's Wort, have been shown to interact with conventional medicines. One safety precaution in particular has not made its way into the herbal canon. Treatments for rheumatoid arthritis, for example, include apple cider vinegar baths, ginger tea and black onion seeds (black seeds from onions or seeds from black onions?). Patients are allowed to wash down said seeds with ginger tea while sitting in a cider bath. Polypharmacy at its very worst.

Homeopathy[9]

This is based on a one-off observation by an out-of-favour clinician in the nineteenth century. Samuel Hahnemann noted that eating cinchona bark (personally) caused fever. Malaria causes fever. Cinchona bark (quinine) helps malaria. Ergo substances which cause the symptoms suffered by the patient will help those symptoms. 'Like treats like' (*similia similibus curantur*).[10] Strychnine will help vomiting, chips will help obesity, a poke in the eye with a sharp stick will help the symptoms of glaucoma ...

Clearly at some stage the apparent lunacy of this struck Hahnemann, so he suggested (OK, he may have said this right from the start) that you use very small quantities (it'll work with the chips). Very, very, *very* small quantities. *Succussion* of the active material – 1:10 dilution with some talented shoogling – would be repeated on a small quantity of the resultant solution. And again. Perhaps 20–30 times. This very dilute[11] preparation would then be used, having been made *more* potent by this process.

---

[8] In similar fashion to the world of science, where many 'heretics' such as Copernicus met a sticky end for attacking the conventional wisdom that the Earth was the centre of the universe. In the world of medicine similar conventional wisdom is now only to be found with respect to London.

[9] The more traditional spelling 'homoeopathy' is now less often used, and signifies that the user is an enthusiast.

[10] I prefer 'like will be treated by like'.

[11] Those of you with a passing knowledge of Avogadro's number will have spotted that a 10^{-30} solution (*30x*) of, say, strychnine will contain only one molecule of strychnine in every 2000 litres (perhaps just as well). Homeopaths are aware of this and claim the water molecules themselves are affected by the succussion and thus somehow maintain the beneficial effects. It is unclear whether this was very much an afterthought when the apparently irremediable flaw in their story was brought to their attention ... 'oh, well ... actually ... now I remember ... he *did* have the gun with him in the swimming pool ...'

Though one or two isolated studies suggest that there could be more to it, most authorities put any benefit from homeopathy down to the placebo effect. Patients are treated very well. Their stories are meticulously taken and the treatments are geared precisely towards their symptoms, rather than towards any non-specific 'disease' title – which in some ways is an improvement on many a practitioner's approach.

Cynical Suggestion No. 1   Homeopathy is a useful way of treating with placebo in a caring and supportive fashion non-seriously-ill patients who would otherwise never accept such management.

Acupuncture

Traditional Chinese acupuncture is based on the concept of the 'cool' Yin and the 'fiery' Yang present in all things – including the organs of the body, where the constant flow of '*qi*' keeps the balance right.

It is difficult to think of this as anything but nonsense, but that doesn't mean that acupuncture can't work. Many remedies that are tried for one reason turn out to work for another. Gold was first used in rheumatoid arthritis to treat the underlying infection[12] – and we still don't know why it does work. Bromide was used in epilepsy because all epilepsy sufferers were thought to be hyp*er*sexual and bromide reduces this (castration was another treatment used as recently as the nineteenth century). Subsequent work suggests that epilepsy sufferers are hyp*o*sexual (though drugs and parental dominance in the inculcation of morality may contribute to this), but the drug proved to be the first ever effective treatment because of its inhibitory effects on the brain.

Allying modern medicine to acupuncture is tricky. The 'gate theory of pain' and other ideas on endorphin release may go some way towards explaining its effects,[13] but most acupuncture trials appear in journals of 'traditional medicine' – where analysis of variance of immunoglobulin and complement values, and *t*-tests demonstrating significant reductions in C-reactive protein, sit alongside observations that the treatment 'dispels wind and cold and removes dampness' in patients with RA (a disease of *bi* – blockage in the flow of *qi*[14]). However, a number do suggest that it might work.

One day I'll get round to the definitive study – comparing 'classic' acupuncture (using the charts of 'spinal warmer' channels, etc.) vs. just jabbing the needle at the sore bits.

Reflexology

Pretty girl manipulates your foot. Feel better? There's a surprise.

---

[12] Yes, I know – not only is RA not an infection, but also gold doesn't treat infections – but it *was* thought of as a treatment for tuberculosis. 'It works in TB, so it might work in rheumatoid' was clearly either crazy or genius. And if we now find (as we will one day) that infection *does* set off RA ...?...

[13] Though who is to say that this would be *correctly* explaining its effects?

Copper bracelets

A favourite of arthritis sufferers. They 'read about it in a magazine'. A recent issue of a patient self-help group journal carried an 'article' by a patient who was self-helped by these ... so was her brother ... and her friends (did they *all* have arthritis?) ... 'and it's so good we'll offer to sell you one ...'

I'm not always convinced that patient self-help group journals are a good thing.

Copper bracelets with magnets

Well, at least you won't lose them.[15]

Diets

Clearly, some people may have some symptoms worsened by particular foods but most diets espoused in books and the like are simply ways of making money from selling books and the like. They may be contradictory – 'established' remedies for arthritis include (1) avoiding all citrus fruits and (2) olive oil and lashings of orange-juice – but this does not deter them.

Food sensitivities are another favourite. Genuine food allergies exist, but the idea of an allergy is often hit upon for no good reason. Fortunately the sort of diseases for which people avidly seek explanation in 'food allergies' are usually the sort of diseases you can happily leave to their own devices.

Chiropractic/osteopathy[16]

Chiropractic was invented by DD Palmer (1845–1913; Iowa), though the idea of spinal control over diseases elsewhere in the body goes back to Hippocrates (much earlier – not Iowa). He made his name with a successful cure of a janitor's deafness (this is Palmer, not Hippocrates – I'm not sure how Hippocrates made his name, though he was one of the first to use willow bark to ease pain and inflammation) by spinal manipulation. Patient reports suggest that everyone who attends an osteopath will be told they have a malalignment of the spine and will then have their backbone crackled like a line of toppling dominoes which will make them feel better for a while. Chiropractic and osteopathy are tolerated by most medics, though lingering doubts over potential injury to the patient tend to ... linger.

---

[14] A knowledge of which word is particularly frustrating, as most authorities refuse to accept its use in Scrabble.

[15] Hot-off-the-press footnote. Ingenious paper just out which compares proper magnetic bracelets with ordinary bracelets with *bracelets having enough magnetism to lift pins and so fool patient into thinking they are proper* ... and ... the proper bracelets seemed to work best!! ...

[16] These two disciplines do differ, but since this difference is only known to enthusiasts, it would be detrimental to your career for you to learn it.

9

Endocrinology

Endocrinology is for losers. It would be doing you a disservice if we even pretended it was worth having a proper section devoted to this specialty, as we must obliterate any leanings you may have in this direction. And the reason for this is:

Cynical Tip No. 41   Endocrinologists do not do well in the private sector.

And the reason for this is ... you don't need them. Endocrinology is all down to numbers. There is no requirement for any expertise or experience, as the numbers give you the answer.

- Your sugar's up, you've got diabetes.
- Your thyroxine's up, you've got thyrotoxicosis.
- Your thyroxine's down, 'go to' (oooooh ... tricky!) ...:
  - your TSH is up, primary hypothyroidism
  - your TSH is down, pituitary disease.

There's none of the 'considered opinion' so characteristic of other specialties. No '... rheumatoid factor is positive, but I think this is a red herring as clinically you've got ...' or '... your angio is normal, but your chest pain does sound ischaemic, so what might be happening is ...'
  No.
  The tests define the disease. So any specialty opinion is superfluous.

History

Tiredness

Once they mention 'tiredness', just do all the endocrine tests. There's no point in enquiring after polydipsia, polyuria, 'what sort of weather do you prefer?' (I ask you, *what sort of weather do you prefer?!!*) when everybody knows you're just going to *do the tests*. If their T_4 is up, it doesn't matter *what* weather they prefer, you'll decide they're thyrotoxic. If their plasma glucose is 45 mmol/l, then the absence of a family history of diabetes isn't going to change your diagnosis.

Fatigue

See 'tiredness'.

Run-down

See 'fatigue'.

Dizzy spells

See 'tiredness', 'fatigue' and 'run-down'. They may suggest an endocrine problem, particularly if they occur on standing, especially in the morning. Postural hypotension. The frequently underlying hyponatraemia is usually caused by drugs rather than by a pituitary or adrenal problem, but it gives you an excuse to ... *do the tests.*

Increasingly large hands and feet

No acromegalic patient ever actually complains of this (well, maybe some).

Examination

All endocrine signs are bogus. Like our previous analysis of clubbing, they are defined retrospectively once the diagnosis is known. 'Remember that really ugly patient I told you about last week ... turns out it was hyperendohorm syndrome facies ...'

Cynical Tip No. 42[1]   In general it's worth assuming that any ugly patient in the exam has an endocrine diagnosis. Ugly examiners, meantime, are simply an occupational hazard and any increased likelihood of their being endocrinologists has yet to be proven (statistically speaking).

The only worthwhile sign in endocrinology is tachycardia/bradycardia (thyroid), but since 90% of the world takes beta-blockers, its usefulness is severely diminished.

The only tricky sign in endocrinology is postural hypotension. Classically the mistake we make is to take the blood pressure with the patient lying down, then take it immediately after they stand up – whereas the cognoscenti know to wait three minutes before taking the second reading. All very well, but since no one can convince me that the reason I suddenly go all woozy if I get out of bed too fast in the morning is that three minutes later my blood pressure is about to drop ...

---

[1] Amazingly, we find that the question of life, the universe, and everything is: *How many Cynical Tips are there?* It only just occurred to me that almost all are in the later part of the book – clearly CVS, respiratory and gastrointestinal specialities have 'harder' signs than neurology and rheumatology.

I tend to take a second reading immediately after the patient stands up (have the cuff on) and another one 2–3 minutes later. If either shows a pathological drop, I think that's significant. What constitutes a 'pathological drop', of course, varies according to sources. Mainly because you can't tell. A systolic drop of >20 mmHg, or a diastolic drop of >10 mmHg has the advantage of being easy to remember (though this diastolic figure might be a bit over-sensitive).

The only fun sign in endocrinology is the delayed reflex recovery in hypo-thyroidism. This just *has* to be performed at the ankles and just *has* to be done in the time-honoured fashion with the patient kneeling on a hard-backed chair, with their ankles dangling over the side. The effect of a sharp tap to the Achilles' tendon is enthralling.

Management

This involves equally straightforward use of numbers.

If there are low levels of something (thyroxine, glucose, growth hormone …) – give them some.

If there are high levels of something (thyroxine, glucose, growth hormone … see how limited this is?!) – give them something that'll stop them making it.

While all of the above ensure that endocrinologists are the only people at our cocktail party who wouldn't mind being mistaken for a rheumatologist,[2] they do drive quite nifty cars (endocrinologists *are* allowed to drive cars – but not to be front-seat passengers – in case the driver falls asleep at the wheel). While their medical prowess is unusable, their ability with figures (and copious free time) allows them to make major killings on the Stock Market.

---

[2] Assuming either might be invited to one.

10

Haematology

'**What is this patient's haemoglobin?**'
A Play in Two Acts

Act 1: A hospital ward round *c*.1980

Consultant:	What is this patient's haemoglobin?
JHO:	Nine-point-three, sir.
Consultant:	Mmmm ... and what's the MCV?
JHO:	One hundred and twelve.
Consultant:	Mmmmmmm ... B_{12} and folate been done?
JHO:	The folate's normal, but the B_{12}'s not back yet.
Consultant:	?
JHO:	It's not back from the lab ...
Consultant:	??!
JHO:	The patient just came in yesterday ... and I've not ... and ... and ... I'll go and see if I can get the result.

Act 2: A hospital ward round *c*.2000 +

Consultant:	What is this patient's haemoglobin?
PRHO:	I dunno.
Consultant:	What's this patient's MCV?
PRHO:	I dunno.
Consultant:	... What is this patient's *name*?
PRHO:	I dunno. I don't work here. I usually work in Ward 16.
Consultant:	This *is* Ward 16.
PRHO:	What? I thought Ward 16 was a surgical ward.
Consultant:	This *is* a surgical ward.
PRHO:	(*looks at watch*) Gosh! Is it February already?

APPENDIX 1

Best ever medical joke

This guy was struggling with horrible pains going right up his left side and down his left arm. Really sore. Really horrible. Totally random times.[1] He went to see his GP. 'I've got these horrible pains going up my left side and down my left arm.'[2] GP examines him. Can't find anything. Refers him to rheumatologist. Patient sees rheumatologist. 'I've got these horrible pains going right up my left side and down my left arm.' Rheumatologist can't find what's wrong (*plus ça change*) and refers him to see a *neuro*logist. An appointment is made by phone and the patient is sent an appointment with a *uro*logist. 'I've got these horrible. ...' Serendipity! The urologist has seen this before.

'I've got good news and bad news. What do you want first?'
'The bad news.'[3]
'I've no idea what causes this.'
'And the good news?'
'I know how to cure it.'
'Hooorah! ...'
'Oh now I remember, there's bad then good then more bad news.'
'?'
'It's only helped by ... castration.'
'That's OK – I'll do anything to get rid of the pains ... what's "castration"? ...'

After an explanation has been given, the offer is declined. Three months later, however, the pains are so bad he can't take it any more.[4] He goes back to the urologist ... signs the consent form ...

Afterwards – the pains are *gone*. The operation was a success.[5] Two weeks later, the pains are still gone. But ...

But ... *for some reason*, he just doesn't feel ... happy. He's depressed. So he does what he's always done to brighten himself up – goes off to buy a new suit. The tailor's measuring him up ... inside leg ... our guy is a bit ... embarrassed. Hope he doesn't notice ...

'And on which side does sir dress?'
'What?'

---

[1] Not important to the joke – but shows we're still alert to asking the right questions.
[2] So, not cardiac ischaemia, then.
[3] Always the correct choice.
[4] He doesn't 'complain bitterly', since these pains are really painful.
[5] OK, a bizarre statement, but this is a *story*.

'Which side do you dress on?'

'What does that mean?'

The tailor tuts. 'When you wear your trousers, which side do you hang your
... you know! ...?'

Total embarrassment for our man. Does he really have to tell his tailor everything?

'Why? Does it matter?'

'Why, sir, of course. If you dress on the left and I make you trousers to
dress on the right ... you'll get these horrible pains right up your left side
and down your left ...'

APPENDIX 2

Litres per minute. L/min. $L\,min^{-1}$.

Index